MORINGA MATTERS

By
Dr. Howard W. Fisher
&
Steve Wilson

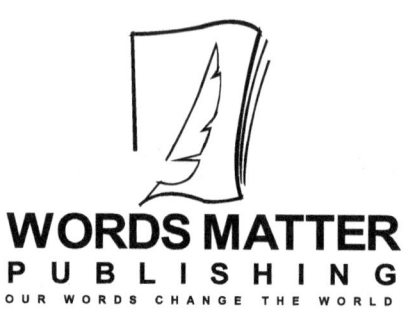

© 2018 by Dr. Howard W. Fisher & Steve Wilson. All rights reserved.

Words Matter Publishing
P.O. Box 531
Salem, Il 62881
www.wordsmatterpublishing.com

No part of this publication may be reproduced, stored in a retrieval system, or transmitted in any way by any means—electronic, mechanical, photocopy, recording, or otherwise—without the prior permission of the copyright holder, except as provided by USA copyright law.

ISBN 13: 978-1-949809-21-3
ISBN 10: 1-949809-21-8

Library of Congress Catalog Card Number: 2018967996

The impossible takes about 120 days, miracles slightly longer

Names of Moringa Around The World

Kannaeng doing, Murunkak-kai, Malunggay, Horseradish tree Chum Ngay, Drumstick tree, Ben aile, Sajna, Mlonge, Nebeday, Manrangon, Benzolive, Jeringa, Dandalun, Angela, Aceitoso, Bamboubamamoer, Moringa, Coliro, Sitachini, Cenauro, Aceite, Goma, Saijan, *Árbol del ben*, Ben, Morango, Mother's Best Friend, Radish tree, Bèn ailé, Benzolive, Moringa, Ben oléifère, Arbre radis du cheval, Behenbaum, Calcita, Behenussbaum, Flügelsaniger, Palo de Tambor, Palo blanco, Bennussbaum, Pferderettichbaum, Sàndalo ceruleo, Acácia branca, Cedra (Brazil), Marungo, Moringuiero, Muringa, Hoja de sen, Chuva de prata, Cedro, Chinta Borrego, Macasar, Moriengo, Marenque, Moongay, Noz de bem, Orengo

There are more than 400 names for Moringa oleifera. Obviously, this plant has made an impact around the world.

TABLE OF CONTENTS

Preface vii
Preface Continued.. xi
Foreword xv

PART I   The Foundation 1

CHAPTER 1
Why Another Health Book?.. 3

PART II   The Science 7

CHAPTER 2
Why Moringa? 9

CHAPTER 3
Genetic Modification 55

CHAPTER 4
Inflammation 75

CHAPTER 5
Obesity 95

CHAPTER 6
Aging 147

CHAPTER 7
Toxins Out Nutrients In 'Dirty Work'...................................179

CHAPTER 8
The Science of Exercise: Uncovering the Facts 185

CHAPTER 9
Protein and Exercise 191

CHAPTER 10
Optimizing For Peak Performance 197

PART III   Moringa Applied 205

CHAPTER 11
So Now What? 207

CHAPTER 12
"THIS AIN'T JEOPARDY" But your life may be in it! 211

CHAPTER 13
Who wants to be a "Health-o-naire?"
Moringa-naire? 253

Bibliography 267

About The Author 301

PREFACE

Our words matter because our lives matter. All of them. What we do matters including how we communicate it to the rest of the world. That's where Words Matter Publishing's slogan comes in: "Our words change the world." Words mean things so we must think carefully before we speak or write because we will be held accountable for them all. With that in mind, we boldly, unapologetically put forth "Moringa Matters."

Does Moringa REALLY Matter?

Well, "let's start from the very beginning"...as Julie Andrews famously sang, "a very good place to start. When you read you begin with A, B, C; when you want health you begin with..."

Well, where do you begin actually? To answer that question, I must start by telling why Moringa matters to me. I must confess I am a "certified organic health nut." But it was not always so.

To make a long story short, I was once growing up overweight and unhealthy. One day, I got sick and tired of being fat, sick and tired. I began reading health publications when I was about 17 years old and started to implement diet and exercise changes. That wasn't always easy growing up in Owensboro, Kentucky—the "barbeque capital of the world"—

which also may just be the "fat, sick and nearly dead" capital or at least close. Suffice it to say, it wasn't easy, but I was able, by the grace of God, to overcome my own health challenges as I learned and continue to learn as much as I can about how to be healthy.

However, in addition to not being easy, it was never cheap either. I used to spend a small fortune at the health food store buying supplements for a growing family (now of 7). That's when I came across a video from one of my health heroes, Ty Bollinger, the best-selling author of *Cancer Step Outside the Box*" and producer of amazing health documentaries among other notable accomplishments in the world of wellness. He was discussing the amazing health benefits of a plant named Moringa oleifera. Ty said at the time it might have been the most important video he had ever sent to his subscribers because it offered a way to get the most nutritional bang for your buck by taking just ONE plant. "WHAT?! ONE PLANT?!" I was floored. Could this really be true?

I had to find out. So I reached out to Ty via e-mail which led to a phone call and a lengthy discussion about this little-known plant which I couldn't even pronounce properly at the time. Ty was very humble and gracious and gave me a wealth of information about the plant. Then he went a step further. He got me on the phone with some guy in Canada who just happened to know a little bit about Moringa.

Of course, saying that Dr. Howard Fisher knows a little bit about Moringa is like saying that Bobby Fischer knew a little bit about chess. Fischer didn't invent chess, but he did arguably more for the game than anyone before or after him. Dr. Fisher didn't invent Moringa but he likewise has done as much or more as any other mortal to shed light on this gift from God. A world-renowned health lecturer, Dr. Fisher is known as an "anti-aging guru." He is the author of 20 books on health, and this one is his fourth on Moringa oleifera. So not only can he pronounce it and spell it, he can tell you about everything you could possibly want to know about it—what it is, what it does, how it does it and why it matters.

You paid a price to buy this book, but there's a much greater cost that you will pay if you read this book without a goal. Your time is your most precious asset. Don't waste it. Don't waste it on a book that won't add value to your life. Don't waste it by passively listening to a health lecture or passively reading a book that contains life-saving information. You must be as actively engaged in reading as the authors were in writing. That's what we believe. That's why we wrote this book.

We, as the writers, demand from ourselves the best. In the years leading up to writing this book, we have asked the hard questions and not rested with superficial answers. We demand the best for our own health and for the health of our families which is why we have taken our time to write this book. Spoiler Alert: We believe that Moringa is the best source of nutrition that God has put on His good creation and that is why we believe MORINGA MATTERS.

But that's about what we believe. We don't imagine you will believe it just because we say so. We don't presume you will believe simply because of all the articles and information cited in this book that agrees with our opinion. Nor do we expect you to agree with our conclusions based on the many testimonials you will read from satisfied Moringa users. We ask that you be as scrupulously demanding in your reading as we were in researching and writing. We expect you to ask the difficult questions and don't rest until you get a satisfactory answer even if that means doing your own follow-up research which is another reason for the plethora of endnotes. If you do all that and are still unsatisfied with the answer, feel free to visit Moringadoctor.com and even contact us for more information as I did with Ty Bollinger when I first heard him mention the plant.

WARNING: "There's a monster at the end of this book!" I love that book also, but I'm not referring to loveable furry old Grover. I'm talking about the monster that confronts us all each time we are confronted with information that can save or enhance our lives. There are truths that are sometimes hard to take in because they require us to make serious changes which can be difficult and/or costly. Well, the truth is the truth whether we like it or not or whether we choose to follow it or not. So the question we ask now and more pointedly later, if you arrive at the same conclusions as the authors of this book, are you willing to make changes accordingly? If not, perhaps you should put the book down now.

Methinks I hear a Dr. Fisher interjection here—"Did you really just write that?! Let them keep reading. You never know when the lightbulb is going to switch on for someone. I mean, look at you, Steve. How many times have I had to tell you something before you finally got it?"

OUCH! Ok, whether you're curious or serious, you've been warned so without further ado…let me introduce you to Dr. Howard Fisher.

Steve Wilson

PREFACE CONTINUED...

I would like to thank all the individuals who were involved in the research used to advance the health of mankind. This, for the most part, is a thankless undertaking. I would like to thank those who freely gave their testimonial evidence about their health and the subsequent changes that occurred as a consequence of making nutritional decisions that involved *Moringa oleifera*. There will be those that choose to ignore this information and those that choose to accept the information and my best wishes go out to both factions.

Despite the fact that a major portion of disease was once believed to be based on genetic predisposition, the completion of the human genome study in 2003 has allowed researchers to reveal that the opposite is true. According to Professor Helena Baranova, "Eighty-five to ninety-six percent of all disease is due to environmental causes."[1] The impact of Professor Baranova's statement is based on her expertise in genomics, the study of the human genome, and in fact, her findings should make us realize that we have to become more aware of the environmental challenges to our health.

My friend Russ Bianchi loves to explain a diversity of seemingly inexplicable phenomena with the following quote referencing Ockham's Razor, "Invariably the simplest answer tends to be the correct one," as suggests. "The simple answer, in this case, is the industrialized, processed, chemically refined, and genetically modified food and beverage chain, along with a tsunami of harmful drugs, is killing us. We are overfed, undernourished, and over-drugged."

Food no longer works! If it did, we would be able to use it to keep our bodies functioning properly, decrease the incidence of disease [2] [3] [4] and furthermore we could use it to provide the nutrition needed to function at optimal states (at peak performance). Scientists, doctors, and inventors are all diligently looking for the key to understanding the mechanisms and multiple functions of food in order to improve our physiology and quality of life. Many professional athletes have already uncovered the secret and of course, having any edge in professional sports can help you all the way to the bank...the health benefits may just be a tremendous bonus.

Lately, there has been more research into nutrition and *Moringa oleifera*, and I would like to opine on these intertwining issues for your benefit. Remember that this is a plant that the US National Institute of Health and Medicine, an official agency for the United States government, has affirmed Moringa can "arrest, reverse, and cure, over 300 different diseases and disorders."[5]

I hope you enjoy my ranting and raving. This book will contain excerpts, abstracts, articles and some testimonials. All testimonials have been sanitized to protect the identity of the provider. Do not expect to understand all of it because there will be a number of abstracts drawn from PubMed in the original jargon but there will always be commentary for impact.

Hopefully, it will be an interesting read because I try to look at all the literature that I can in this field. Currently, there are more than 500 papers on *Moringa oleifera* on pubmed. gov. I urge you to investigate the links and visit the websites for any of the papers or articles that interest you. There will be repetition which hopefully will serve to reinforce the basic knowledge about this plant and how it will benefit us.

Moringa oleifera is the most phytonutrient dense plant on the planet and provides the physiological needs for the body to maintain optimum health and therefore seek homeostasis for all parameters.

Do nothing, and your life may go on subject to the whims of others and enter entropy, however, the decision to take effective action in a proper sequence enabling a proven, predictable formula will allow you to manifest significant change. Continue in those actions, and it will only be a temporal relationship before you achieve the results of that formula: extropy. Which would you rather have? Either can be in your future it all depends on you and the philosophy of the mentor you choose.

We have a good idea what are the factors in major diseases and the solutions to these are absent from our food chain. For decades we have known that oxidative stress plays a major role in the onset and etiology of diseases such as cancer, atherosclerosis, diabetes, and neurodegenerative disorders but have not really made this common knowledge.[6] [7] [8] [9] [10] Inflammation seems to play a fundamental role in the incidence of so many chronic diseases and their progression, and it has direct ties to atherosclerosis, coronary artery disease, and cardiovascular disease. [11] [12] [13]

Moringa Oleifera may, in fact, be the world's best kept nutritional secret. *Moringa oleifera* may be the world's most phytonutrient dense plant on the planet. *Moringa oleifera* may be the plant that possesses the ability to positively transform the current status of health and decrease the incidence of disease around the world. *Moringa oleifera* will improve the performance and results of those who choose to exercise for whatever reason.

Hippocrates adage about giving the body what it needs and the body will correct itself has been deranged by the fact that environmental issues have caused such a great amount of chronic disease that this is not possible. I have taken the liberty of modifying Hippocrates' adage, "Give the body what it needs, and the body will repair itself to the best of its ability. If you give the body Moringa, those abilities increase."

For those of you who care about the truth! It is not about the fight. It is not about being right. It is about sharing what you know to be true. Time heals all wounds by proving their other disingenuous agendas. As Mahatma Gandhi said, "First they ignore you, then they laugh at you, then they fight you, then you win."

Dr. Howard W. Fisher

FOREWORD

"Never confuse activity with results," was the advice I was given at the age of 12, by an eminent scientist, who became a prominent globally recognized Nobel Laureate. This advice never leaves my brain as a formulator.

The science of sports kinesiology and measurable results has advanced exponentially on this globe in the past three decades.

Many major successful sports brands, including several energy bar and drink brands, have been formulated by me. Said another way, I know what works and what does not.

However, it really grates me to see efficacious formulations or products dumb-downed, or intentionally blocked from use, by greedy, stupid, and unscrupulous economic marketers, once delivered for production or distribution. Yes, this happens far too often, but products that truly deliver, in the end, win.

Dr. Howard W. Fisher has once again achieved 'GOLD' with this cutting-edge treatise on the true and proven benefits from efficacious *Moringa oleifera*, with impeccable research sightings.

As I write this brief forward, Dr. Fisher's pondering about the use of Moringa oleifera in the Olympics is in fact reality. In both the 2012 and 2016 Games, dozens of medal winner athletes have contributed to their performances using enzymatically bioavailable and completely safe, as well as efficacious sports and muscle building, moringa brands that I formulated. The same is also true in the pre-collegiate, collegiate, and professional ranks of athletes in many sports, including sanctioned world record holders.

Dr. Fisher is absolutely correct that much can be corrected and improved through telomerase enzyme enhancement, which enzymatically standardized and fully bioavailable *Moringa oleifera* does far better than any other single or combined, protocols, I have ever measured.

You could go far and wide, at much greater time and expense, with far less results, and not get even a fraction of empirical truth provided in this succinct and 100% factual book.

Russell M. Bianchi, Co-Founder,
Speech Morphing INC

PART I

The Foundation

CHAPTER 1

Why Another Health Book?

Why another "health book?" Why any book for that matter? But we wrote another in a vast ocean of health books, and the question is a resounding WHY? The question for you is WHY will you read it? I've gone to and helped to organize many health lectures in my life, and I've discerned there are essentially two types of people who attend. Some are curious, and others are serious. Some merely want to learn the next new idea in the world of health while others seek to significantly advance the state of their health and lives. Which one are you? And it's ok if you are the former. It's ok if you bought the book out of curiosity. However, we the authors will ask the same from you at this point as we would from those who are serious about boosting their health.

Whether it's a health lecture or book, you must ask yourself why you are attending or why you are reading. Everybody's got another theory, a new idea and many of them are good. I've benefited from many of the books on wellness that I've read and been able to apply a lot of what I have learned which I believe has led me to better overall health. Then one day I was sitting down to do my own personal health checklist, and I realized, "wow, this is hard." I can't possibly do everything on this list every day. I understood at that point what I should have grasped long ago, but sometimes we have to get hit in the head over and over before we decide it's high time to "KEEP IT SIMPLE STEVE!"

But can obtaining great health be simple? If it was easy, everybody would do it, right? Many of us who are health-conscious can seem like zealots to our extended family and circle of friends. We are often labeled "health nuts" and perhaps even ridiculed for our "beliefs." We then have a tendency to become puffed up by the health knowledge we have acquired and can look down on those who make less than optimal choices regarding their own well-being. I know I've done it. I've been on my high horse more times than I care to remember. I have been far too ready to condemn and write off for good those who didn't agree with me. If you didn't believe like I did, you might as well be burned in effigy along with Ronald McDonald and Col. Sanders for killing the masses with food-like substances.

For those who are similarly health-minded, it can sometimes be just as difficult getting along. We end up engaging in the "my health guru can beat up your health guru" rhetoric that gets us nowhere fast except living on our own private health island. But is that ok? "I'm healthy and happy and content on my island. You stay on your island. I won't bother you, and you don't bother me." No! It's lonely for one. More importantly, what if you have a better idea that would help me? I should at least be humble enough to listen. By the same token, what if I know something that could benefit you as it has helped me? As part of obeying the sixth commandment—"Thou shalt not kill"—I have a positive duty to not only not kill you, but if it's in my power to help prolong your life and enhance your health, I should seek to do it. That is also in keeping with my Lord and Savior's command to "love your neighbor as yourself."

So I sat for many days on my private health island wondering how do we connect with others? How do we build a bridge which unites us at least in the arena of health? Is what I have worthy of consideration? I could tell you how Moringa has enhanced my overall health but would that be enough to get me on your island for you to even consider bringing a Moringa plant you've probably never heard of on to yours? Perhaps one of my favorite metaphors would be helpful to speak to this central theme of the book.

What's the End Game?
After I squandered a clear advantage and lost a chess game to him, the older and wiser player remarked, "If you don't have an end game, you don't have a game." He went on to say that the Russians actually start with the end game. I think the analogy is apropos here. If we think of the concept of health as a chess game what is the objective?

Dr. Fisher already mentioned there were a lot of pre-existing agendas out there and he said his agenda is to get you to start caring about your own health and that's a great place to begin. From there, we have to narrow the scope significantly as there are many components to health. The purpose of this book is not to entertain every arbitrary and capricious speculation—from the 99-year-old chain-smoking granny to the 44-year-old man who dips in the lake in the winter—as to how to obtain some real or conceived measure of health and longevity.

The purpose of this book is to ask one very important question. That question is not, can Moringa help me live forever? No, it can't. If that answer disappoints you, I refer you to another book—the Holy Bible. The purpose of this book is not to point out all the health problems we are facing especially in North America thanks to GMOs and the SAD

(Standard American Diet). That's in here, but it's not the main point.

Our clearly-defined end game for putting forth this book is that we want to put the power back in the hands of the people. We want to ignite a health revolution and paradigm shift in the way communities and individuals define healthcare from one of disease management to one of disease prevention. We want YOU to take personal responsibility for your own health. We want you to join the army of health freedom-fighters and then go recruit others in this very serious conflict.

What is our weapon of choice for this health revolution? Maybe there's more than one. But is there one BEST, most powerful weapon in the battle for getting optimal nutrition in the face of overwhelming health risks especially here in North America where I write this at 9:37 a.m. CST on November 6, 2018? Ok, I hear my "inner Dr. Seuss" demanding…

The time has come
The time is now
Just ask the question
I don't care how!

Is there a plant given by a loving and wise Creator which is able to replace the missing amino acid profiles and supply an enzymatically active, bioavailable, antioxidant-rich, anti-inflammatory rich, natural source of nutrition?

OR perhaps even simpler: Is there a nutritional BEST bang for the buck for the whole living, breathing, dying world?

Want to find out? Keep reading as Dr. Fisher presents the science of Moringa…

PART II

The Science

CHAPTER 2

Why Moringa?

'Here, There, and Everywhere'

I thought that this book would be different and that it would be the sort of eye opener to make people realize that they should look into the information being disseminated by the diversity of pre-existing agendas. It seems every faction has an agenda and my agenda is to educate you to the point that you care about your health. More than thirty years of treating patients and listening to the plethora of reasons for lack of compliance has made me realize that I can only offer guidance and that any form of implementation in a free society rests with you.

I live in Toronto, Canada and we have one of the largest busiest highways in the world, Highway 401, which has more than sixteen lanes at some points, and there is always traffic. This services the metropolitan population of approximately seven million people. My responsibility to the patient is to give advice, and if I were to warn them not to play in the middle of this highway because they might get hurt, I have carried out my responsibility. If they do and they get hurt, I have done all that I can do. If they were to run into a problem and I also gave advice which resolved the problem it is very much the same thing.

This book will be exactly that, but in this case, please feel free to read the articles, many of which are taken directly from the source and footnoted so you can easily find them. There are many opinions expressed here, both my own and those of hundreds of other researchers and authors so feel free to accept what you will and disregard the rest. You may find many facts repeated…let the impact sink in because these statistics are important as they reflect how things have escaped our control.

It is apparent that if there was a 'State of the Food Chain Address', that you would want to make changes to improve your health with this knowledge. I have been lecturing about the broken food chain for a while so now let's hear it from some others.

I came across this quote from Nick Pineault about how fruits and veggies are on the qualitative decline, "because agriculture has selected certain genetics to maximize sugar content and resistance to certain pests—all while decreasing the soils' quality with abusive farming practices—most veggies and fruits grown today now contain way fewer nutrients than 50 years ago."

In a 2009 article, 'Declining Fruit and Vegetable Nutrient Composition: What Is the Evidence?' Donald R. Davis states that the average vegetable found in today's supermarket is anywhere from 5% to 40% lower in minerals (including magnesium, iron, calcium, and zinc) than those harvested just 50 years ago.

What about transit time, storage time and facilities? What are they doing to your produce? According to Martin Lindstrom, author of the book "Brandwashed," the average supermarket apple is 14 months old. 80% to 90% of adults in the US don't get enough vitamin D 34% of men & 27% of women don't get enough vitamin C Around 74% of adults don't consume enough iodine 68% of Americans are magnesium deficient 40% of all adults are deficient in vitamin B12.

Here is what the CDC had determined and how many deficiencies apply to you or someone that you know.

The Centers for Disease Control and Prevention coordinate data into a report called the National Health and Nutrition Examination Survey (NHANES) highlighting nutrient deficiencies in the population. The top deficiencies are viewed from the perspective of dietary intake, absorption and "endpoint" metabolism. End-point metabolism is a definitive index of the nutrient requirement levels based on physiology.

Vitamin C (Antioxidant)
Indications include: weakness, fatigue, gums bleed easily, nosebleeds, bruising easily and increased healing time

Sources: leafy green vegetables, fruits and of course *Moringa oleifera*.

Vitamin B-12
Indications include: mood problems, memory problems, mental fatigue, and poor concentration, irritability, poor circulation, and decreased REM sleep

Sources: eggs, milk, cheese, milk products, meat, fish, shellfish and poultry, and Moringa oleifera.

Vitamin D
Indications include: poor blood sugar stability, chronic pain, gait and clumsiness issues, immune system problems and hormonal issues. Vitamin D is activated in your skin and muscles and functions better with ample magnesium.

Sources: some fish and *Moringa oleifera*, other than that Vitamin D is not available from dietary sources.

Magnesium
Indications include: constipation/irregular bowel activity, indigestion, irritability, muscle cramping (cal-mag imbalance), tremors, decreased enzymatic activity (zinc is also very important here).

Sources: plant-based foods (chlorophyll), such as *Moringa oleifera*, nuts and seeds, green algae, avocados, and leafy green vegetables.

Omega Essential Fatty Acids
Indications include: depression, hormone imbalance, decreased immune system function (fibromyalgia and C.F.S), decreased energy stamina, neurological problems, poor concentration

Sources: *Moringa oleifera*, coldwater fish, flax, and walnuts.

How many people have you spoken to who have told you that they do not need supplements because they eat well? The statement should be amended to' they think that they eat well' because they do not actually realize how damaged the food chain actually is. Humans were meant to survive by breathing air, drinking fluids and eating food and in this manner, the bulk of the population should be healthy. Since most people do not get ill from a lack of oxygen or dehydration one might correctly assume that the food chain is not supplying proper nutrition and therefore the body cannot deal with the environmental factors that cause disease.

With a US population of over three hundred million there are over 700 million chronic diseases...who is healthy? Allegedly eating well is a band-aid solution that in fact is like trying to repair your road with duct tape. Reality should be setting in now, and you should look for the best source of nutrition. I know a plant that covers all the bases.

Many of us are aware of the idiom about the cat that swallowed the canary and the interpretation of this idiom indicating that feeling that one had had a very successful venture. From my perspective, in determining a nutritional approach to move away from the chronological clock, we are always seeking the proverbial 'canary.' What is the best nutrition we can possibly put in our body? In the 1990s there was a big buzz over spirulina and chlorella, another member of the blue-green algae family. These are tremendous nutrition sources as you will see in the following paragraphs from an article just out today but the fact of the matter is that they cannot even come close to the nutrition contained in *Moringa oleifera*.

"Elderly folks suffering from anemia or age-related immune system deterioration could see dramatic improvements with regular supplementation of spirulina, blue-green freshwater algae with an extensive track record of health promotion and disease mitigation. Researchers from the Division of Rheumatology, Allergy and Clinical Immunology at the University of California, Davis, (UCD) learned this after testing the effects of spirulina on a group of seniors with either or both of the two conditions and seeing positive results."

"Participating in the study was a cohort of 40 volunteers, each of whom was 50 years of age or older with no previous history of major chronic illness. Each participant did, however, report having suffered from some form of anemia or immunological dysfunction, also known as immunosenescence, meaning he or she was in need of regular treatment. In this case, researchers wanted to test whether or not a nutrition-based approach centered on spirulina would bring relief to the volunteers."

Now these algae have chlorophyll, protein, iron, vitamins, and minerals and they would be a good supplement if you were not aware of *Moringa oleifera* which has more of everything and a lot more antioxidants, Omega 3 FAs, chlorophyll, anti-inflammatory phytonutrients...well, in fact, pretty much everything you need....

Now you will understand why providing an enzymatically-alive version of *Moringa oleifera* to your body brings about such remarkable changes. The food chain is broken, and it is time to give your body the nutrition it needs.

Thanks, blue-green algae for holding the fort until the troops arrived.

Natural Cures for Mankind

Research has suggested that there may be natural cures that are effective against much of what is plaguing mankind. I found this quite interesting...and yes there are more than turmeric and D3....

This accidental finding reached by scientists further shows the lack of real science behind many 'old paradigm' treatments, despite what many health officials would like you to believe. The truth of the matter is that natural alternatives do not even receive nearly as much funding as pharmaceutical drugs and medical interventions because there's simply no room for profit.

In fact, some research shows that current methods are just not working,

"These results delineate a mechanism by which genotoxic therapies given in a cyclical manner can enhance subsequent treatment resistance through cell on autonomous effects that are contributed by the tumor microenvironment."[14]

http://www.cureyourowncancer.org/study-accidentally-finds-chemo-makes-cancer-worse.html#sthash.HCCSC95C.dpuf

If everyone were using turmeric and vitamin D for cancer (better yet cancer prevention), major drug companies would lose out.

So there are natural cures and we need them

So it is sort of official...we can no longer take the approach of treating cancer...we have to get preventive. I have been on this preventive approach for thirty years, and now they realize the importance of diet and environment. I think perhaps the introduction of a phytonutrient dense plant would be the perfect intervention.

"A new report from the World Health Organization warns that cancer rates around the world will experience a 57 percent surge over the next 20 years." That would mean cancer diagnoses would rise from an estimated annual total of 14 million to 22 million. Deaths from cancer are also expected to rise during the same period, from 8.2 million deaths a year to 13 million.

The WHO's World Cancer Report says that healthcare providers around the world will not be able to address the problem by simply treating cancer patients. In fact, the report argues that current cancer treatment costs—estimated at an annual $1.16 trillion—are already hurting major world economies.

Instead, the organization advises that governments focus on prevention and early diagnoses.

"We cannot treat our way out of the cancer problem," Christopher Wild, director of the International Agency for Research on Cancer, told CNN. "More commitment to prevention and early detection is desperately needed in order to complement improved treatments and address the alarming rise in cancer burden globally."

Do you not think that it is extremely interesting that most people on the planet have never heard of *Moringa oleifera*. Do you think that there may be other agendas in place? The *Moringa oleifera* tree aka the horseradish tree, drumstick tree, benzolive tree, kelor, marango, mlonge, moonga, mulangay, nébéday, saijhan, sajna or Ben oil tree (over 200 names), has been used by the ancient Hebrews (Moses as directed by the Creator) Romans, Greeks and Egyptians. How is it possible that the most phytonutrient dense plant that had been in use for 5000 years vanished? Perhaps it is time to look at preventative measures.

One of those preventive measures should be to include polyphenols in your diet. I may be somewhat redundant, but there is so much information supporting this fact that it is important that people understand why Moringa oleifera works in the capacities related to complete nutrition and anti-aging. This may help give you more insight.

Papers such as Sreelatha et al. (2009) Antioxidant Activity and Total Phenolic Content of Moringa oleifera Leaves in Two Stages of Maturity and Moyo et al. (2012) Polyphenolic content and antioxidant properties of Moringa oleifera leaf extracts and enzymatic activity of liver from goats supplemented with Moringa oleifera leaves/sunflower seed cake will make all the information below relevant. In a nutshell, there is a 30% reduction in mortality if you have a dietary intake of polyphenols and from the above papers, you know that *Moringa oleifera* has a high polyphenol content.[15][16]

High Dietary Intake of Polyphenols Are Associated With Longevity

Oct. 9, 2013—It is the first time that a scientific study associates high polyphenols intake with a 30% reduction in mortality in older adults. The research, published in Journal of Nutrition, is the first to evaluate the total dietary polyphenol intake by using a nutritional biomarker and not only a food frequency questionnaire. Research is signed by Cristina Andrés Lacueva, Montserrat Rabassa, and Mireia Urpí Sardà, from the Department of Nutrition and Bromatology of the UB; Raúl Zamora Ros (ICO-IDIBELL), and experts Antonio Cherubini (Italian National Research Centre on Aging),

Stefania Bandinelli (Azienda Sanitaria di Firenze, Italy) and Luigi Ferrucci (National Institute on Ageing, United States).

Read the whole article:

http://www.sciencedaily.com/releases/2013/10/131009111025.htm#!

I thought I should emphasize the importance of what Moringa brings to the polyphenol portrait. Polyphenols are naturally occurring compounds that are present in vegetables, fruits, coffee, nuts and a number of natural foods. They generally have beneficial functions: antioxidant, anti-inflammatory, anti-carcinogen.

Dr. Raúl Zamora Ros, the first author of the study on mortality reduction based on phenolics intake published in the Journal of Nutrition, points out that "results corroborate scientific evidence suggesting that people consuming diets rich in fruit and vegetables are at lower risk of several chronic diseases and overall mortality." In conclusion, the research proves that overall mortality was reduced by 30% in participants who had rich-polyphenol diets (>650 mg/day) in comparison with the participants who had low-polyphenol intakes (<500 mg/day)."[17]

I guess to be totally direct, all the polyphenols you need daily are available in two ample servings of *Moringa oleifera*.[18]

What to Look for in Your Moringa

I receive about fifty phone calls and two hundred emails every day. It is not an uncommon sight for me to be walking down the fairway to hit my next shot, smartphone in hand. Yes, I bend time, and it works for me. Every day, because those in the know are growing in numbers so rapidly, I receive several calls with the exact same question. Which *Moringa oleifera* is the best? The answer is obviously one that complies with the following critical criteria:

There are so many differences in what Moringa versions may be made available in health food stores or anywhere else and the Moringa oleifera that I prefer. Let us start with the fact that the best moringa is one specific varietal of thirteen species and scores of varietals which is the most potent.

Organically grown...either you grow hydroponically, or you are able to control all the farms in the district so no windblown pesticides and fertilizers whereas most are grown anywhere. The best available source controls all the plantations in the district to ensure that no one is using any pesticides or fertilizers in the district.

Hand picked and sorted. Not including just leaves but the fact that many growers buzz down the tree and mix all the parts together bark and all (some even include the roots). The best version that I have seen involves a proprietary formula involving five different Moringa components and does not include bark or roots (which can be toxic)

Enzymatic activity degrades above 104 F. The most efficacious form of *Moringa oleifera* plants are **shade-dried** (most growers save money by putting plants into driers which lose their enzymatic activity due to temperatures above 104 Fahrenheit) Also ultraviolet (UV) light will degrade the enzymatic activity of many plants and growers that use these techniques have far less effective plants.)

Handling and shipping. Long shipping times when the plants are exposed to the environmental factors may decrease the potency and effectiveness of any phytonutrient unless proper care is taken. Most cannot afford to vacuum pack and shipped to the United States for processing in an FDA approved facility that manufactures at pharmaceutical grade quality. (Food grade processing for most others is all that is required, and the criteria are the same as your local restaurant on some table in a back room not in a completely sterile facility that uses clean rooms.)

So the unknown Moringa mulch put into one of these capsules is not just leaves (and leaves themselves cannot compare to the proprietary formula of the best version that I have seen) but perhaps dried bark and roots and then the question is how much goes into each capsule...a maximum of 500 mg. ONE pouch of the proprietary Moringa formula that I personally advocate contains more than one ounce. Now I know I will still get this question every day, but now you know.

How To Get The Most Out Of Your Moringa

I have noticed that there seems to be a concept that needs to be clarified...competitive nutrient absorption. Do not eat at the same time you consume your Moringa. Whenever I am asked the best manner in which to ingest *Moringa oleifera*, I suggest a 45-minute window on either side with no other food. This will allow the phytonutrients in Moringa unrestricted access to the sites for nutrient absorption with no competition from other less beneficial foods. First thing in the morning is a great time. There are only a limited number of absorption sites and why would you want competition in allowing your body to receive the best nutrition to allow optimal physiological function. 45 minutes will allow other foods or *Moringa oleifera* to pass through your stomach and small intestine.

Restoring Health... Testimonial

In March of 2012, I had little energy and was couch bound as soon as I arrived home from work, exhausted. Even though I had been taking supplements of all kinds, eating well and exercising regularly, I still lacked energy and was unable to lose weight. I jokingly used to say to my work-out partner "I must have a tapeworm because I'm doing all the right things, but I'm exhausted and can't shed a pound or an inch off my midsection."

My insurance broker heard about my health challenges and explained she had a great whole food supplement that would "Naturally" increase my energy levels AND reduce weight. I was willing to try anything, so we literally did a "drive by" and she gave me a box of a proprietary formula of *Moringa Oleifera* along with some information about this tree that I had never heard about.

I had been struggling with my weight, high blood sugars, high cholesterol, hypothyroidism, a hormonal imbalance, severe sleep apnea, and depression/anxiety for many years. My doctor recommended putting me on medication for diabetes and cholesterol in addition to already being on anti-depressants and hypothyroid medication. I begged him to let me try something natural first and recheck my blood levels in three and six months. He agreed to allow me to give it a try and so began my *"Moringa Oleifera"* healing journey.

As I learned more about *Moringa Oleifera*, I was impressed by the long list of nutrients that were readily available in a 100% Bio-Available natural plant form that I could take once or twice a day mixed with water. This had everything I was looking for! Weight loss, skin care, detoxification and all of the nutrients required by the human body to achieve perfect health

I love information on health, so I quickly went to hear one of the doctors speak about the research of *Moringa Oleifera*. It seemed that finally my prayers had been answered. I started taking it, and within a few days, I felt an increase in my energy levels, a clearer head, and a feeling of well-being. Within three days, I passed both flukes and other lovely parasites from my body. One week later I passed a five-inch tapeworm…they say better out than in. I also knew that it probably was only part of the tapeworm, so I continued cleansing.

Within two weeks I dropped 12 lbs., lost inches off my waist and felt better than I had in years. I was even able to get a good nights' sleep. All without changing my diet or exercise routine. After three months of taking Moringa, I added some other proprietary Moringa products into my regimen and found that I slept better and lost more weight.

Six months later my sugars came down from 15 to 4.5, my cholesterol returned to normal, my eyes are clearing, and my doctor is weaning me off of my Antidepressant medication. My doctor was pleased that I took responsibility for my own health and he even read the book that I had about Moringa. After taking "Moringa Oleifera" for one year now, I notice my body continually reshaping, shedding more fat and my energy levels have never been so high. I even had someone guess my age at 39! I am 50!

I seem to be reversing my age every day and returning my body to the best health that I can with the nutrition in this plant. I truly believe the *Moringa Oleifera* tree is a gift to heal the planet!

Energy and Wellbeing Testimonial

For the last three months, I have been taking a proprietary Moringa formulation. I started taking four sachets daily, and I have now cut back to only three. One of the first things I noticed right after starting was that I felt such an unusual sense of well-being, not just in areas where I was feeling symptoms but everywhere. I still have this feeling! My whole body works much better, and I have a lot more energy despite a heavy workload and an extremely busy time-tight daily schedule. I do actually sleep less than before. I like to wake up an hour before the alarm goes off in the morning, and know that I am well rested!

I also got rid of my troublesome psoriasis-like eczema which I have had for years, and that no cortisone cream prescribed by my doctor or otherwise has managed to affect. Even my hair has been affected by this Moringa formula, and it grows more quickly than before, and it has become richer and thicker.

I am so glad that I started with Moringa and hope many more people are discovering the great health benefits that the product can provide. I recommend it to everyone around me because it actually works.

Follow The Health Ranger & You Will Live Longer

Have they known that plants offer the solution to health? You be the judge.

Nearly 100 years ago, the AMA began removing nutritional education from medical schools in America. Medical doctors would no longer understand anything about using food as medicine (or be allowed to suggest it), and all midwives, Native American herbalists, and natural healers would be referred to in medical journals as "quacks." The Western Medicine philosophy would soon come to be that no food in the world could ever heal a human being or cure any disease or disorder; in fact, only pharmaceuticals and vaccines would ever be able to make that claim (legally) and get away with it, whether in peer reviews, medical and science journals (JAMA), scientific "studies" or labeled as such on products. (http://www.naturalnews.com/)

Currently, it is illegal for any food, herb, tincture or superfood product to say that it cures anything, yet medications advertised on TV since 1997 can say they treat all kinds of diseases and disorders, even though the side effects are horrendous, some of the time including internal bleeding and suicide. (http://www.naturalnews.com/)

Mother Nature, on the other hand, has a CURE for everything and also offers prevention and immunity for everything under the sun. Nutritionists and Naturopathic

Physicians will tell you all day that organic fruits and vegetables are the key to healing and living a healthy life. A plant-based diet can heal nearly any health problem, and the body is like a machine that fires "on all cylinders" when given the correct fuel. Take this knowledge and be on your way to health freedom and natural living, where you have lots of energy, rarely ever get sick, can think critically all the time, can be spiritual and independent and take care of your family! Follow Natural News and track the truth. Learn and grow from it. Don't eat cancer. Don't drink cancer. Be organic.

Learn more:

http://www.naturalnews.com/042688_natural_medicine_cancer_cures_government_agencies.html#ixzz2j1u0haNo

Vitamin A and Reversing Cancer
Were you looking for another reason to make *Moringa oleifera* part of your daily regimen? Retinoic acid, a derivative of vitamin A which is found plentifully in *Moringa oleifera* has been shown to transform pre-cancerous breast cells back into their normal, healthy state.

Retinoic acid can be produced in the body by two sequential oxidation steps that convert retinol to retinaldehyde and then to retinoic acid. Medical oncologist, Professor Sandra V. Fernandez of Thomas Jefferson University, and her research team evaluated the effect of retinoic acid on four types of cells, each one representing a different stage of breast cancer: normal, pre-cancerous, cancerous, and a fully aggressive model. Results showed that the retinoic acid had a marked effect upon the pre-cancerous cells, not only making them look like healthy cells again, but also reverting their genetic signature back to normal. However, cells that were considered fully cancerous did not respond at all to retinoic acid, thus suggesting that there may only be a small window of opportunity for retinoic acid to be helpful in preventing cancer progression. In addition, only one concentration of retinoic acid (about one microMolar) produced the anti-cancer effects – lower concentrations had no effect, and higher concentrations produced a smaller effect. After the success of this study, the researchers are hoping to determine whether the amount of retinoic acid required can be maintained in an animal model.[19]

Most of us in the west would find it almost unbelievable that worldwide, an estimated 670,000 children die annually from Vitamin A deficiency.[20]

Moringa has natural energy... the others are a lot of bull!

If you thought you knew what was in that energy drink... think again. Thanks to the Daily Buzz Live for the following eye-opening article.

Energy Drinks Contain Ingredient Extracted From Bull Urine And Semen. A study done by Longhorn Cattle Company tested some of the top energy drink brands such as Red Bull, Monster, etc. What they found might leave your stomach in a knot. They found that the drinks do, in fact, contain bull semen. Taurine is the ingredient that has come under fire. Taurine is named after the Latin Taurus, which means bull. It was first isolated from ox bile in 1827 by Australian scientists Friedrich Tiedemann and Leopold Gmelon. It is often called an amino acid, even in scientific literature, but it lacks a carboxyl group it is not strictly an amino acid. Taurine is present in bulls livers, semen, and urine. One thing is certain, the taurine used in energy drinks such as Red Bull is taken from these sources.

Taurine found in energy drinks is a byproduct of bull testicles, it is considered not to be vegetarian-friendly. The ingredient is taurine, a naturally occurring substance that is present in bull bile and breastmilk. The video shows how this ingredient is extracted from the bulls. It was filmed by an employee of the company that supplies this ingredient to the various energy drink company. The video was then Leaked, leaving to us this secret they have tried to keep quiet for so long. The employee was later fired for violating company policy.

http://dailybuzzlive.com/archives/4763#sthash.K5x2Eo2a.A6kmF6Qi.dpuf

If you want energy plus a lot more, there is nothing that compares to the natural energy provided by the most phytonutrient dense plant on this planet...*Moringa oleifera*.

What is in there? How Much Do I Need?

I was doing a Q & A webinar last night, and I was asked a question that I receive so often that I have to count to ten before my response leaves my lips. What is in there? How much of this does it have? I took 5 minutes to answer this question last night because I had to establish the frame of reference that apparently NO ONE with the diverse range of products available has or could even have the ability to compare the answer to, and that involves the consumption of products that are enzymatically alive. Most are dead.

Dead products cannot contribute much of what they contain to the body and cause the body to use a lot of energy in the creation of enzymes. The proprietary formula of Moringa that I advocate has 25 g of Moringa when hydrated, and the concentrated about 50 g. I said on the call that people who ask these questions really do not understand plant-based nutrition...they understand chemical-based extracts that your body can only absorb 10% to 25%.

Dosage is not based on what's in the plant...it is based on how much you weigh and how toxic you are. Your body will extract 90-95% of the nutrition in an enzymatically alive plant because that is what your body was designed to do...extract nutrition, when available, from a food source. The more natural the food source, the more nutrient dense the food source, the easier it is. The obvious answer is not to look for numbers assigned to chemical nutrients, but basically to put the whole food plant-based nutrition into your body and let your body sort it out. Remember that the determining factors are size and toxicity.

Where are you getting your minerals?

Studies that compared the mineral content of soils today (1992) with soils 100 years ago (1892) found that agricultural soils in the United States have been depleted of eighty-five percent (85%) of their minerals.[21]

Do you think it is getting better or worse...twenty-two years later?[22]

"Research suggests that taking vitamin B supplements may help reduce the risk of stroke. Xu Yuming, of Zhengzhou University and colleagues analyzed 14 randomized clinical trials with a total of 54,913 participants.[23] All of the studies compared B vitamin use with a placebo or a very low-dose B vitamin for a minimum of 6-months. Results showed that taking supplementary vitamin B lowered the overall risk of stroke by 7%. However, taking supplementary vitamin B did not appear to affect the severity of strokes or the risk of death from stroke. The authors concluded that vitamin B supplementation significantly reduces stroke risk by lowering levels of the harmful amino acid homocysteine." [24]

So the above study shows that people who take B vitamin supplements reduce the risk of stroke by 7%. Vitamin supplements are absorbed from 10% to 25% whereby plants are absorbed 90% to 95%. *Moringa oleifera* contains copious amounts Vitamins B1, B2, B3, B6 & B7. A little-known fact is that vitamins do not work without minerals and Moringa oleifera contains significant quantities of minerals enabling the vitamins to function more optimally.

What might the finding of that study be when conducted using a far more potent source of B vitamins? The fact that the literature contains many papers pertaining to cardiac benefits and Moringa intake is not a coincidence.

What Do You Really Know about Magnesium?

Estimates indicate that approximately 60% of the population does not get enough magnesium daily and intake has declined by 50% in the last century.

Magnesium, like zinc, plays an integral role in hundreds of physiological functions. From bone health, DNA synthesis, energy metabolism, enzyme activation, expelling toxic metals, immune system function, muscle relaxation, workload duration, and regulating blood pressure, magnesium is one of the most common intracellular ions. Both of these minerals are plentiful and easily absorbed from *Moringa oleifera*.

Findings have shown a decrease in hyperactivity, "In the group of children given 6 months of magnesium supplementation, independently of other mental disorders coexisting with hyperactivity, an increase in magnesium contents in hair and a significant decrease of hyperactivity of those examined has been achieved, compared to their clinical state before supplementation and compared to the control group which had not been treated with magnesium."[25]

One of the reasons we see a profound change in ADD and ADHD children taking *Moringa oleifera* is the combination of Zinc and Magnesium found in this phytonutrient dense plant. "The improvement achieved in ADHD children with the use of zinc sulfate appears to confirm the role of zinc deficiency in the etiopathogenesis of ADHD."[26]

The Most Effective Way to Get Your Magnesium

Enzymatically-alive green plants such as *Moringa oleifera* contain chlorophyll and chlorophyll plays a critical role in human health as it is virtually identical to the hemoglobin (red blood cells) in our bodies with the exception of the core molecule (magnesium instead of iron). Magnesium will attempt to displace most of the heavy metal toxins and cause them to be forced out of the body.

Magnesium Deficiency

Hypertension, Osteoporosis, Heart disease, Muscle spasm, poor glucose metabolism, sleep disorders

Adequate Magnesium

Decreased diabetes, decreased muscle spasm.

Life Just Got Better...Testimonial

I have been using a proprietary *Moringa oleifera* formula for twelve months and lost 15 pounds in the first two months. I also gained muscle mass and lost 18 inches, and all these changes occurred at the age of 67.

    I had regained the weight I'd managed to keep off for about ten years, and with the combination of low energy, feeling negative, moral and physical fatigue, muscular pain, I was just drained. My immune system was malfunctioning, and I was getting one cold or flu after the other and had problems with my lungs and coughing. I looked like an old woman.

    After a few months of using the proprietary formula, I started using some moringa products on my face. My hair and nails have improved, my skin is firmer (even face, neck and upper arms), my immune system has greatly improved (no colds since last February). These results can even be seen in my blood tests. My digestive system and elimination function better too. Best of all I have my energy back and have a brighter outlook...I am even socializing more since I feel better. I see improvements happening on an ongoing basis, and at present, one year later I can truthfully affirm that I have gotten younger and have improved memory.

NEED SOME ZINC?

Oregon State University Study

SAYS THAT YOU DO

Zinc deficiency mechanism linked to aging, multiple diseases

10-1-12

CORVALLIS, Ore.—A new study has outlined for the first time a biological mechanism by which zinc deficiency can develop with age, leading to a decline of the immune system and increased inflammation associated with many health problems, including cancer, heart disease, autoimmune disease, and diabetes.[27]

The research was done by scientists at the Linus Pauling Institute at Oregon State University and the OSU College of Public Health and Human Sciences. It suggests that it's especially important for elderly people to get the adequate dietary intake of zinc, since they may need more of it at this life stage when their ability to absorb it is declining.

About 40 percent of elderly Americans and as many as two billion people around the world have diets that are deficient in this important, but often underappreciated micronutrient, experts say.

The study was published in the Journal of Nutritional Biochemistry, based on findings with laboratory animals. It found that zinc transporters were significantly dysregulated in old animals. They showed signs of zinc deficiency and had an enhanced inflammatory response even though their diet supposedly contained adequate amounts of zinc.

When the animals were given about ten times their dietary requirement for zinc, the biomarkers of inflammation were restored to those of young animals.

"The elderly are the fastest growing population in the U.S. and are highly vulnerable to zinc deficiency," said Emily Ho, an LPI principal investigator and associate professor in OSU School of Biological and Population Health Sciences. "They don't consume enough of this nutrient and don't absorb it very well."

"We've previously shown in both animal and human studies that zinc deficiency can cause DNA damage, and this new work shows how it can help lead to systemic inflammation," Ho said.

"Some inflammation is normal, a part of immune defense, wound healing and other functions," she said. "But in excess, it's been associated with almost every degenerative disease you can think of, including cancer and heart disease. It appears to be a significant factor in the diseases that most people die from."

As a result of this and what is now known about zinc absorption in the elderly, Ho said that she would recommend all senior citizens take a dietary supplement that includes the full RDA for zinc, which is 11 milligrams a day for men and 8 milligrams for women. Zinc can be obtained in the diet from seafood and meats, but it's more difficult to absorb from grains and vegetables—a particular concern for vegetarians. "We found that the mechanisms to transport zinc are disrupted by age-related epigenetic changes," said Carmen Wong, an OSU research associate, and co-author of this study. "This can cause an increase in DNA methylation and histone modifications that are related to disease processes, especially cancer. Immune system cells are also particularly vulnerable to zinc deficiency."

Research at OSU and elsewhere has shown that zinc is essential to protect against oxidative stress and help repair DNA damage. In zinc deficiency, the risk of which has been shown to increase with age, the body's ability to repair genetic damage may be decreasing even as the amount of damage is going up.

Medical tests to determine zinc deficiency are rarely done, scientists say and are not particularly accurate even if they are done. The best approach is to assure adequate intake of the nutrient through diet or supplements, they said, especially in the elderly. Even though elderly people have less success in absorbing zinc, the official RDA for them is the same as in younger adults. That issue should be examined more closely, Ho said.

Levels of zinc intake above 40 milligrams per day should be avoided, researchers said, because at very high levels they can interfere with absorption of other necessary nutrients, including iron and copper.

These studies were supported by the National Institutes of Health and other agencies.

Moringa oleifera is an extremely phytonutrient dense plant and an excellent source of bioavailable easily absorbed zinc when it is from an enzymatically alive plant. "Furthermore, restoring zinc status via dietary supplementation reduced aged-associated inflammation. Our data suggested that age-related epigenetic dysregulation in zinc transporter expression may influence cellular zinc levels and contribute to increased susceptibility to inflammation with age."[28]

Glutathione

I have had a great deal of positive feedback on this particular blog, and I was asked to expand it…. Some people watch TV, but for me, TV is background noise while I read journal papers. I thought I might just appeal to the interesting side of being a researcher, so you know why I answer questions the way I do. Someone once asked me how many papers I have read about *Moringa oleifera*...it is a number with at least three zeroes. The mechanisms for phyto-nutrition may never be known. No one will pay for the significant research costs involved to determine the mechanisms for a plant that is not patentable. If you want to know why some of the things that happen to people who consume *Moringa oleifera* regularly, the answers can be found in the literature. In this paper, 'Fakurazi et al. (2008) *Moringa oleifera* prevents acetaminophen induced liver injury through restoration of glutathione level. That should be an eye-opener.

Now the reason this paper is interesting is because a few other companies talk about nothing other than glutathione and *Moringa oleifera* just maximizes these levels by itself as a natural plant. 'The level of glutathione was reduced with APAP treatment at 1.56 ± 1.19 lmol/g. When the rats were pretreated with MO, both treatment doses (200 and 800 mg/kg) have significantly elevated the level of glutathione in the liver compared to the group receiving APAP only, at 2.59 ± 1.60 and 2.65 ± 0.21 lmol/g, respectively. Pretreatment of 200 mg/kg and 800 mg/kg MO have significantly ($p < 0.05$) protected the liver from hepatocellular damage.' [29]

Translation: The mouse genome study was completed in 2002. The human genome study was completed in 2003. If you want to know why mouse research is so predominant for human testing is because the mouse genes and human genes are 99% identical. Mouse testing allows an extremely valid translation of effects. *Moringa oleifera* elevates glutathione levels to the extent that the glutathione levels protect the liver.

Every system in the body is affected by the status of the glutathione system, most predominantly the gastrointestinal system, the immune system, the nervous system, and the lungs. Glutathione is the primary self-made antioxidant produced by the cells, combating free radicals (ROS) and donating an electron to the electron cascade keeping other antioxidants active. It is highly functional in most metabolic and biochemical reactions (making and repairing DNA, protein, prostaglandin synthesis, iron metabolism, amino acid transport, and enzyme activation Glutathione regulates the nitric oxide cycle) which is essential for proper physiological function but can be challenging if unregulated and in combination with zinc a major factor in sexual arousal. As we can see from the above paper, *Moringa oleifera* elevates glutathione levels to the extent that the glutathione levels protect the liver.[30] Whoa...think about this. How much more does *Moringa oleifera* give than the significant elevation of glutathione levels?

Return To The Living Testimonial
My cousin, a 35-year-old former drug addict, called me up and when we met, he was skin and bones and very ill. He has been drug-free for several years. He was in such poor condition that he was only able to keep down rice and water and had seizures daily leaving him so fatigued that he had to lie down most of the day. I sent him my proprietary Moringa formula in early April. He started with 1/2 a packet of Moringa increased to 1 after a few days. One week later I received the message : "This Moringa has made me feel a lot better. I have recovered masses in just one week. This is amazing stuff. Now I start the day with one sachet of the proprietary formula and adhere to a very strict diet. "

After one month: "I am so totally happy with this Moringa. It is absolutely fantastic...I feel better and better with each passing day. I am slowly but surely coming back to life...I feel so blessed to be able to see family and friends get back their life!

Adaptogens? *Moringa oleifera* is the most potent

Here's another piece of the Moringa puzzle. Many of us have heard of Ginseng, Maca, and Reishi mushroom (not so many about Moringa yet). These are all well-known adaptogens and in many countries accepted as the most beneficial thing to put into your body in these places. In 1958, two Russian doctors, I.I. Brekhman and I.V. Dardymov defined an adaptogen: "A substance that is innocuous and cause minimal disorders in the physiological functions of an organism, it must have a nonspecific action, and it usually has a normalizing action irrespective of the direction of the pathological state." The bottom line translation of this is give your body what it needs, and your body will respond.

I have written two books on Reishi mushroom, the number one superior herb in traditional Chinese medicine (TCM). Being categorized as a superior herb in TCM means there is no limit on the consumption, and that a person may have as much as they want or require. Since the bulk of China is not within the climatic range of Moringa growth, they chose Reishi. Good plant...but not close.

Most people have not heard about *Moringa oleifera*...yet. I am also the author of two books about *Moringa oleifera* which from my research goes far beyond the capabilities of any other adaptogen on this planet, and that includes Reishi. Give the body what it needs, and the body will use the nutrition it receives to optimize physiological functions.

Chronic Liver Inflammation Testimonial

Years ago, in 1998, I was diagnosed with chronic liver inflammation that slowly destroys the liver. After taking a blood test, I was diagnosed with liver cancer in March 2011. After taking a blood test, I was diagnosed with liver cancer in March 2011. I received a CT scan after a few weeks, but nothing could be found. The blood test was also negative. I received no medication. But later in 2012, they gave me a heavy regimen of interferon and a pair of anti-viral medications against chronic hepatitis C, producing similar side effects as chemotherapy. The treatment had to be interrupted due to internal bleeding in both the retina and the stomach. After this procedure, I was far from completely recovered. In addition to the liver disorder, I was floored when I got the diagnosis of chronic fatigue syndrome.

Aside from that, I have had chronic degenerative arthritic back pain for many years, and I was using strong pain medication. I have gone to chiropractors and physiotherapists who only helped for a short time, and I have been living with this pain. I have had joint and muscle pain throughout the body (fibromyalgia), a stroke in 1989, a heart attack in 2001, very high blood pressure and major sleep issues for years which almost turned me into a zombie. I was genuinely distraught and had no idea what more I could do other than die. I thought about this often.

In the midst of all this, an old acquaintance I had not heard from in a while, called. She is a dietitian, reiki master, and healer and she has been desperately searching for years for something that could help me in my hopeless health situation. I knew she was always very skeptical of all forms of 'miracle cures' propagandized by the health food industry, but with this *Moringa oleifera* plant, she was over the moon. I met with her and started taking a proprietary *Moringa oleifera* formula.

And now, six weeks after I started everything has turned upside down, in a very good way. My blood pressure is normal. I sleep at night and feel almost as energetic as when I was young, and I am now 55 years old. Back pain does not bother me anymore! I have just recently checked my liver enzymes, and the previously highly elevated results are falling towards normal. Now I think almost anything is possible—it seems to be a miracle.

And while we mention optimizing physiological functions...how about the immune system

Immune modulation of dried Moringa (powder) in diets for human use and livestock production- Intervention with a diet containing 5% Moringa leaves powder was investigated using a rat model and compared to a 5% common cabbage diet, and a nutrient-sufficient diet without vegetables. After 3 weeks, the preliminary result indicated that the Moringa leaves powder diet lightly reduced blood triglycerides and enhanced immune response due to increased peripheral and splenocyte T-cell proliferation. The preliminary study implies the consumption of moringa leaves powder may increase immune response in nutrient-deficient subjects.

In addition, consumption of nutrient and phytochemical-rich vegetables, like Moringa, leads to a better immune response compared to consumption of vegetables that are rich in fiber but lower in nutrient or phytochemical content, like common cabbage. Moringa should be promoted for greater consumption for human use to improve nutrition and strengthen immune functions.[31]

I wonder if this explains anything? Or everything? What do you think?

Cannot buy your health? Guess again

The expression used to be that you cannot buy your health but people were under the fallacious impression that you could buy food which at one point about eighty years ago may have contained a modicum of nutrition. Apparently whatever nutrition was present in the form of phytonutrients, vitamins, minerals, and all of the other physiological components needed to sustain physiological integrity cannot be found in your local supermarket. This relationship between health and nutrition was the basis for my first Moringa book.

The food chain has been broken, and whether it has been done deliberately or not, the fact remains that it is. More than 200 enzymes need zinc to function affecting every aspect of your health from your skin to your brain and even libido. *Moringa oleifera* contains copious amounts of minerals such as zinc, calcium, iron, magnesium, copper, and many more. Each of these plays a unique physiological role in our health. Over the counter vitamins (poo poo pellets) usually end up untouched in the toilet due to their glycol coatings so they don't work and vitamins need minerals to function. Do you know where you can find both in one plant?

Apparently You Can Buy Health…Testimonial

As a teacher, I was always getting sick with colds and flu. My husband and I recently had full blood work done. The blood test revealed that my husband and I both had high cholesterol. I was low in iron, which I have always been low in iron my whole life. My husband was told that he would have to go on cholesterol medication. He also had a spot on his lung. We didn't want to go on any medication because of the side effects but thought that we might have to.

We were introduced to a proprietary formula of parts of the *Moringa oleifera* tree. Ten weeks after starting this high quality, nutrient-rich, enzymatically alive formula my husband went back for a full blood work again. His bad cholesterol (LDL) was down by 25%, and his good cholesterol (HDL) increased 5%, and the spot on his lung did not get any bigger. The doctor was amazed and was sure that my husband had radically changed his diet, but both of us had not changed a thing except for taking Moringa formula.

Ten weeks later, we both went for another full blood test, and it was amazing. Both of our cholesterol levels are perfect, and my iron level is perfect. The spot on my husband's lung was just about gone completely. The doctor was pleasantly surprised and said that we had the best blood test results that he had ever seen.

While taking this proprietary Moringa formula, both of us noticed that our craving for junk food was decreasing and our food intake amount was decreasing as well. Within 6 weeks, my husband had lost 20 pounds, and I had lost 35 pounds. My husband has lost a total of 35 pounds, and I have lost a total of 65 pounds (size 24 down to a size 10) without feeling deprived or restricted at all. Neither one of us did any exercise, and we ate what we wanted. Our bodies were now craving 'good' food and not 'junk' or 'artificial food.'

We now know that the Moringa is giving our bodies all of the nutrition we need so that we don't have to eat the excess of food with extra calories in order to get the nutrition. Both of us noticed, just within 6 weeks of starting, that our aches and pains have gone away, and we are a lot more flexible. My adult acne has disappeared, and our skin is softer and younger looking. My husband's arthritis has gone away as well, and he is now able to move and work without pain or stiffness. Our eyesight has improved, and the 'cloud' in our brain has lifted, and we can think clearer. We have lots of energy and feel so much younger and more alive. It is nice having energy at the end of our busy days. By the way, my husband is in his mid-60s, and I am in my mid-50s.

Now that the Moringa products are in our lives, we would not be without them, and it is making our quality of life and love for life so much better. It is great jumping out of bed and enjoying life.

P.S.: Our 13-year-old dog was having trouble getting up after sleep, and her eyes were quite cloudy. After one month of the Moringa, her eyes are clear, and her stiffness is gone. She jumps, runs and plays like a young dog again. Her coat is shinier, and she is not shedding as much as she did before. All we do is sprinkle a little of the Moringa proprietary formula on her food in the morning and night.

Moringa and Pregnancy

A common question is about *Moringa oleifera* and pregnancy... should I take the standard vitamin supplements prescribed by obstetricians or real food? I recently talked about the difference in absorption of supplements in comparison with other foods (supplements 10% to 25%, plants 90%-95%). It is well documented that *Moringa oleifera* is the most phytonutrient dense plant on the planet containing more iron than spinach (5.3-28.2 mg vs. 2.7 mg in spinach), more vitamin C than oranges (220 mg vs. 69.7 mg per average orange), and more potassium than bananas (1324 mg vs. 422 mg per banana). The calcium content in the leaves of *Moringa oleifera* is extremely high with a 73% absorption rate and a 59% retention rate, and the oxalate content is one-tenth that of spinach.

Moringa has been shown to double the production of Mother's breast milk whether it is consumed before or after the birth of a baby. I personally know many women taking *Moringa oleifera* who got pregnant, had extremely healthy babies and are now giving *Moringa oleifera* to their babies and perhaps anyone reading this who has had a child or knows a friend or family member who has had a child while taking *Moringa oleifera* will comment below. Now some articles note that *Moringa oleifera* has anti-fertility and abortifacient properties. With the exception of the roots and bark, all parts of the Moringa tree support the mother and fetus nutritionally.

It is well documented that Moringa oleifera is the most phytonutrient dense plant on the planet containing more iron than spinach (5.3-28.2 mg vs. 2.7 mg in spinach), more vitamin C than oranges (220 mg vs. 69.7 mg per average orange), and more potassium than bananas (1324 mg vs. 422 mg per banana). The calcium content in the leaves of Moringa oleifera is extremely high with a 73% absorption rate and a 59% retention rate, and the oxalate content is one-tenth that of spinach.

So now the question arises as to which company supplying *Moringa oleifera* does not contain these two parts of the tree. As the author of two books on *Moringa oleifera*, I have spoken with several companies that provide this product to the public. None of them provide at the level of the product anywhere close to the one I recommend. From their FDA approved facility that manufactures at pharmaceutical grade and vertical control from plantation to consumer, this company knows exactly what is in their *Moringa oleifera* products. I spoke directly to their formulator, and he assured me that none of the formulations that I recommend contain the roots or bark and therefore qualify as excellent nutritional supplementation for pregnant women.

Plant-based nutrition...the obvious choice

It is always appreciated when a group such as the ***PHYSICIANS COMMITTEE FOR RESPONSIBLE MEDICINE*** contributes a quote that captures the essence of many of our nutritional deficits. Thanks for this wonderful quote.

"Sometimes the most elegant solution is the most simple. Why plant-based nutrition? Why not? Why develop heart disease? Cancer? Diabetes? The epidemic of chronic, degenerative disease that is sweeping the western world can not only be stopped; it can be reversed. The power lies in the hands of the consumer, in the choices we make about what to put on our plates."

Dr. Howard W. Fisher & Steve Wilson

Sometimes I get carried away...

Those of you that know me also know that I have done a lot of lectures on nutrition from many different approaches, and sometimes I get carried away and get into it, and suddenly it is two hours later, and the people that left halfway through returned realizing that I wasn't stopping to give them a restroom break. When I lecture about Moringa at least people have stopped asking me what's in there because I show them this:

Amino Acids- Alanine, Arginine, Aspartic Acid, Cystine, Glutamine, Glutamic Acid, Glycine, Histidine, Isoleucine, Leucine, Lysine, Methionine, Phenylalanine, Proline, Serine, Threonine, Tryptophan, Tyrosine, Valine

Anti-Inflammatories- Arginine, Beta-sitosterol, Caffeoylquinic Acid, Calcium, Chlorophyll, Copper, Cystine, Omega 3, Omega 6, Omega 9, Fiber, Glutathione, Histidine, Indole Acetic Acid, Indoacetonitrile, Isoleucine, Kaempferal, Leucine, Magnesium, Oleic Acid, Phenylalanine, Potassium, Quercitin, Rutin, Selenium, Stigmasterol, Sulfur, Superoxide Dismutase, Tryptophan, Tyrosine, A, Thiamin (B1), C Ascorbic Acid, E Alpha Tocopherol, E (Delta Tocopherol), Zeatin, Zinc

Antioxidants- Alanine, Alpha-Carotene, Arginine, Beta-Carotene, Beta-sitosterol, Caffeoylquinic Acid, Campesterol, Carotenoids, Chlorophyll, Cholesterol, Chromium, Delta 5-Avenasterol, Glutathione, Histadine, Indole Acetic Acid, Indoleacetonitrile, Kaempferal, Lutein, Methionine, Myristic Acid, Palmitic Acid, Prolamine, Proline, Quercitin, Rutin, Selenium, Superoxide Dismutase, Threonine, Trytophan, A, B Choline, B1 Thiamin, B2 Riboflavin, B3 Niacin, B6 Pyroxidine, C Ascorbic Acid, E Alpha Tocopherol, E Delta Tocopherol, E Gamma Tocopherol, K, Xanthins, Xanthophyll, Zeatin, Zeaxanthin, Zinc–Carot-Alpha-Carotene, Beta-Carotene, Chlorophyll, Lutein, Neoxanthin, Violaxanthin, Xanthophyll, Zeaxanthin

Cox 2-Inhibitors- Caffeoylquinic Acid, Kaempferol, Quercitin, Omega 3

Nutrients- Omega 3, Omega 6, Omega 9, Fiber, Flavenoids, Folate, Glutamine, Glutamic Acid, Iodine, Iron, Isoleucine, Leucine, Lutein, Lysine, Magnesium, Manganese, Methionine, Molybdenum, Phenylalanine, Phosphorus, Potassium, Protein, Threonine, Tryptophan, Valine, A, B Cholinbe, B1 Thiamin, B2 Riboflavin, B3 Niacin, B6 Pyroxidine, B12, C Ascorbic Acid, D, E, Zeaxanthin, Zinc, E Alpha Tocopherol

Fatty Acids- Arachidic Acid, Bechenic Acid, Gadoleic Acid, Lignoceric Acid, Myristic Acid, Omega 3, Omega 6, Omega 9, Palmitic Acid, Palmitoleic Acid, Stearic Acid, Kaempferol, Quercitin, Selenium

Glycosides- 4-Alpha-L-Rhamnosyloxy-Benzylglucosinate, 4-Alpha - L-Rhamnosyloxy-Senzylisothiocynate, Niazinin A, Niazinin B, Niaziminin A, Niaziminin B, Niazimicin, Rutin

Sterols- 28 Isoavenasterol, Betsitosterol, Brassicasterol, Campestanol, Campesterol, Cholesterol, Clerosterol, Delta-5-Avenasterol, Delta 7, 14 Stigmastanol, Delta 7 Avenasterol, Ergostadienol, Stigmastanol, Stigmasterol

Minerals- Calcium, Chromium, Cobalt, Copper, Fluorine, Iron, Lithium, Manganese, Magnesium, Molybdenum, Phosphorus, Potassium, Selenium, Silicon, Sodium, Sulfur, Vanadium, Zinc, Zirconium

Phenols- Caffeoylquinic Acid, Alpha Carotene, Beta Carotene, A, D, E Alpha Tocopherol, E Delta Tocopherol, E Gamma Tocopherol, K, Biotin. B1 Thiamin, B2 Riboflavin, B3 Niacin, B6 Pyridoxine, C Ascorbic acid, Folate

I know I may be evil for doing it that way in a massive list, but people usually realize that this plant is intense. The correct formulation is also enzymatically alive and extremely potent. So do not ask me what's in it. Just ask me how much you need to put into your body.

Everyone's talking about it and you know where to get the best!!

Moringa: Everything You Need To Know About The Newest Superfood

Justin Sedor, Wellness Assistant Refinery[29]

The word "superfood" gets tossed around a lot. It seems like every food is super these days, from pomegranate to chocolate to kale. We're starting to ignore all the marketing noise that cites the presence of "superfoods" in order to distract from a product's high sugar or fat content. So, naturally, we were a bit skeptical when we heard about moringa, a relatively new addition to the superfood pantheon.

So, we did some sleuthing, and it turns out that this one might just be the real deal. *Moringa oleifera*, a tree native to India and the Himalayas but now cultivated in South America and Africa, has been an important food source in some communities for millennia. The tree leaves pack a serious nutritional punch—we're talking high levels of 90 different nutrients, including protein, fiber, calcium, potassium, iron, vitamin C, and vitamin A. But, it's the plant's antioxidant content that has scientists really excited: 46 different kinds, to be exact.

Sounds pretty nifty, right? We're expecting moringa to be one of the breakout nutrition stars of 2014. Right now, though, while you can definitely pick some up at supplement stores in tablet or powdered form (hello, green smoothies!). But, with stats like these, we're thinking moringa won't be a secret for long.

You do know where to get the best, don't you?

Vitamins do not work?

As most of you realize I receive hundreds of inquiries daily, and I do my best to deal with most of them. By now, many of you have seen the Health Ranger's discussion whereby the powers that be are chastising vitamins. Here is my standard response to a question many of you may ask.

Subject: Vitamins in the news.

It would seem that the right hand doesn't know what the left hand is doing. A number of years ago there were a few medical journal articles supporting supplements for some medical conditions (an amazing revelation at the time). I wonder if Big Pharma underwrote this latest study. Do you have a one-line reply to this latest arrow at supplements? It is probable that most people will lump Moringa with Centrum et al. and equate it with a supplement and not a nutrient containing natural vitamins and minerals.

Supplements are generally plant-based extractions and isolations (although often chemical based) and as such are only

10 to 25% absorbed by the body. Being coated with propylene glycol excipient does not help.

Real plants that are enzymatically alive are 90%-95% absorbed and provide the body with a different far more substantial nutritional profile and were not mentioned in this pharmaceutical industry funded study.

Plants versus Pills

All the multi-vitamins out there allege to contain all the vitamins and minerals needed for physiological functions. You should also realize that bio-availability and absorption are two totally different factors and that you will absorb 90-95% of plant-based nutrition which should be complete with minerals whereas only 10-25% of isolates, extractions, adulterated fractions...well you get the idea.

Vitamins do not work without minerals...minerals work without vitamins but not the other way around. So here's what is totally absorbable waiting for you in *Moringa oleifera*.

Moringa Mineral Content

Macro-elements (%)

Calcium 3.65%
Phosphorus 0.30%
Magnesium 0.50 %
Potassium 1.50 %
Sodium 0.164%
Sulphur 0.63 %

Micro-elements (mg/kg)

Zinc 31.03
Copper 8.25
Manganese 86.8

Iron 490
Selenium 363.00
Boron 49.93

And this is just the tip of the iceberg.......the relationship between nutrition and health can be found in my other book!!

As I travel, I notice the current poor health status of a rather significant cross-section of the global population. I am still amazed by the number of poor health choices. There is still a massive amount of work globally for those of us trying to help... try to remember about keeping your equipment functioning at optimal capacity and then providing the raw materials. Most people do not, and it shows in the way that health declines...80% of all the money spent on your health occurs in the last 90 days of your life. It is usually poor choices that lead to this.

A Gift For the Kidney

Those of you in the Nation understand it. Those who have read the chapter in Exodus realize who gave us this gift. The research is overwhelming lately. Eat as much *Moringa oleifera* as you can and allow your body will do the rest. This particular research paper is about the kidney.

Abstract

Present investigation shows that hydroethanolic extract of Moringa oleifera (MOHE) and its isolated saponin (SM) attenuates DMBA induced renal carcinogenesis in mice. Isolation of SM was achieved by TLC and HPLC and characterization was done using IR and (1)H NMR. Animals were pre-treated with MOHE (200 and 400 mg/kg body weight; p.o), BHA as a standard (0.5 and 1 %) and SM (50 mg/kg body weight) for 21 days prior to the administration of single dose of DMBA (15 mg/kg body weight). Administration of DMBA *significantly (p < 0.001) enhanced level of xenobiotic enzymes. It enhanced renal malondialdehyde, with reduction in renal glutathione content, antioxidant enzymes, and glutathione-S-transferase. The status of renal aspartate transaminase, alanine transaminase, alkaline phosphatase and total protein content were also found to be decreased along with increase in total cholesterol in DMBA administered mice. Pretreatment with MOHE and SM significantly reversed the DMBA induced alterations in the tissue and effectively suppressed renal oxidative stress and toxicity.*[32]

There is no better gift than the gift of health.

Intentional Destruction of the Food Chain?

I have been lecturing on the fact that the food chain has been destroyed for many years. The evidence is overwhelming. The Health Ranger, Mike Adams, believes it is by design. *"I have arrived at a conclusion so alarming and urgent that it can only be stated bluntly. Based on what I am seeing via atomic spectroscopy analysis of all the dietary substances people are consuming on a daily basis, I must now announce that the battle for humanity is nearly lost. The food supply appears to be intentionally designed to end human life rather than nourish it."*

This statement is suggestive of other agendas having control of our lives, so how is one to take back control. Back to the paper delivered by Lowell Fuglie fifteen years ago and his commentary then about African malnutrition should be considered now by us, "Moringa added on a daily basis to a child's food, has thoroughly demonstrated its ability to bring about rapid recoveries from moderate malnutrition. But while successfully treating malnutrition is good, preventing it is much better. Malnutrition is brought on by a multitude of causes: lack of education, poverty, famine, parasites, and impure drinking water are but some of them. A program which focuses on correcting micro-nutrient deficiencies alone will not fully eradicate malnutrition until these other causes are addressed. However, as the Moringa project in south-western Senegal has demonstrated, this approach can show very impressive results in reducing the incidence of malnutrition." Now we should add to his list the intentional destruction of the food chain.

Thank You Lowell!

Most people do not know who broke the 'secret' of *Moringa oleifera* to the Western world...his name was Lowell Fuglie working with the Church World Service. In an address in Dar es Salaam, Tanzania in 2001 he revealed some amazing information. You may find this quote about pregnant women interesting..." Women who consume Moringa during pregnancy will have babies with higher birth weights. During lactation, mothers will produce more milk and have increased appetites. Through the project's collaboration with local health posts, successful treatment of malnourished children with Moringa has been well-documented."

Thanks Lowell.

Lyme Disease Testimonial

For the last eight years, I have not felt 100% well. I would wake up each day with what seemed to be a new set of symptoms. One day I would have pain in my hip, one day, pain in my muscles. In 2009 I realized that something was really wrong because I could not remember things that people were saying and I was hurting everywhere and sleeping almost all the time.

I went to my M.D., and he did a blood test that was sent to Igenix Laboratories. The results came back March of 2009, and I had Lyme disease. I was referred to a specialist who put me on high doses of antibiotics for seven months, and I was left with extreme fatigue, forced to take naps twice a day. My body was filled with pain, and I could not carry on a coherent conversation. I was so affected that my Mother was forced to move in with me because I simply could not take care of myself.

On Sept.13.2011 a very good friend of mine called me and asked me to read some information about a plant called Moringa Oleifera. He sent me some of the research that he had uncovered and I went through it from top to bottom. I immediately called him back. "HOW DO I GET THIS PLANT?"

I met with a gentleman the next day, and he gave me some products to try and almost immediately after I started taking it, I knew I had a miracle in my hands. My Mother noticed that I had not had a nap for 3 days, I was speaking clearly, and I had no brain fog. I was excited. The next few weeks saw an even greater improvement and people around me were taking notice. I could actually function.

I had girlfriends asking me what I was doing because I was so different. I shared with them the information, and they too asked how to get this product. The side effect was that as I was feeling better and better and dropping weight. This plant provides total nutrition. It is amazing what can happen when you give your body complete nutrition.

My mother who is 82 years old is also taking the products, and her weight has come down from a size 16 to **a 12. I have dropped 40 pounds since I started. Size 16 to 10 in 6** months! All due to giving my body what it needs. For me, this has been a life-altering experience, and I will continue to share it with everyone because you never know when you will change the life of another soul.

Another Lyme Testimonial

In 1992 when I was 20 years old, I was bitten by ticks and got probably Lyme disease. At that time no one knew much about this disease, and six months after the bite I became paralyzed on the right side. I did not have any thoughts that it could be related to the tick bite. The doctors could not find anything (they still miss this all the time), and I was diagnosed with psychosomatic disorders. The problems progressed, and from 2003, I was 100 % disabled, and then I also suffered from debilitating migraines.

The paralysis lasted for seven years, but all the other symptoms continued including this ongoing constant influenza symptoms which have lasted over 20 years: Always tired, and exhausted and pain all over my body. When I really had the flu, I did not notice any difference except for the fact that with the viral flu my body temperature was high as I had a fever.

I started with the proprietary Moringa formula in February 2014 this year, taking four doses a day. After a week, adverse reactions started to occur. My tongue was white and hairy, and there were black dots on it. I had a metallic taste, headaches and a worsening of my illness. After three weeks on Moringa, all the symptoms began to calm down. I was told that this was a normal detox reaction.

Today, only one and a half months after I started the Moringa proprietary formula, the flu-like symptoms are almost gone. I'm still struggling with pain, but it is better to have pain than not having energy. I no longer have to control everything I do with my will. Before, I had to think about every action every day and talk myself into bearing it, even standing on my legs. I had to always plan my days, so I got enough rest and sleep, enough just to manage to do normal everyday things.

Yesterday I washed the house, baked two cakes, played with and walked the dog before I went to a spinning class for an hour and finished it off with an evening visiting a friend.... Absolutely amazing! I now walk around humming. I still have migraines, but I hope that this too will be better. There is nevertheless a difference of attacks today than in the past. I had a migraine both Sunday and Monday this week but felt perfectly fine on Wednesday. Usually, I am knocked out for several days from a single attack, but Wednesday I washed windows and was in fine form. I have a life again and more every day.

Migraines, Seizures and PMS Testimony

Although I am only 27 years old, I have suffered from debilitating migraine headaches and seizures for the last nine years. These started at the same time when my father died of cancer. These headaches were intense, and the seizures lasted up to three days at a time. I was willing to do anything for relief, so I tried many different medications and treatments, but nothing helped. I seemed to get somewhat better in 2011 until February 2013 when I had another member of my family diagnosed with cancer, From then I was suffering seizures only 4-5 times a month and migraine headaches 3-4 times per week. This was no way to live. My quality of life went downhill with a lot of absence from work, little social life and I was constantly tired. I tried to exercise, but my condition forced me to limit physical activity.

In May 2014 a friend recommended me to try Moringa oleifera and since I have only had one bout of a headache and seizures and it happened when I was out of my proprietary Moringa formulation. Now I'm at work every day. I exercise 3-4 times a week, and I have a new life. Before I really struggled with full-blown PMS; nausea, acne, fever, and severe abdominal cramps and I have always got migraines during my period, and amazingly, they are completely gone. My cramping has been really reduced, and it is not half as much as before. I don´t have to call in sick at work . I have a new life. Healthy eating, regular exercise, healing, and Moringa were the keys to my new migraine-free life! And just to let you know when I had migraines, I had to just lie in the dark, so I lay in the dark room 3-4 days a week for almost 9 years...I am so grateful!

You May Want To Spend A Little Now

My philosophy of health started when playing high school football as a 5' 6" 135-pound wide receiver. I could catch almost anything and had speed HOWEVER at that size your health is always in jeopardy...especially when you are the smallest guy on the field. I remember one drill at practice where all ball carriers had to get used to getting hit and found myself looking at two immense linemen, 240 and 250 pounds respectively, who had dispensed my blocker immediately. I dropped my head and ran...when I woke up on the ground with that circle of stars moving in a clockwise manner; I realized an important fact of life....you are responsible for your own health.

This responsibility never eluded me since I have always sought the best when it comes to health in all aspects: nutrition, exercise, meditation, water quality, air purification, and radiation protection. As most of you will quickly have to adjust your thinking about health care, I suggest that you accept the responsibility for your health and be proactive. Even before the changes to the health care system, 80% of healthcare costs occur in the last ninety days of life.

What happens when the decisions become the choice of others? It has already been demonstrated that no agency will safeguard your health better than you. Those of you in the 'Nation' have already made the choice that will do more for your health in the long term: maximum nutrition. Share this with everyone that you care about for it will change the susceptibility to the environmental factors that shape the health profile demographics of our society.

CHAPTER 3

Genetic Modification

'Pretzel Logic'

People get ready because the change is coming?

Monsanto Has Been Removed And Banned By: Austria, Bulgaria, Germany, Greece, Hungary, Ireland, Japan, Luxembourg, Madeira, New Zealand, Peru, South Australia, Russia, France, and Switzerland!

Is your country on this list? Why Not?

Monsanto claims that GMOs are safe.

This was the same comment made by the tobacco companies back in the 40s and early 50s regarding cigarette smoking.

GMO Corn/Soy Seeds- Fed To Americans But Blocked By China!

U.S. Can Learn From Cyprus Environment Commissioner: National Launching Of GMO-Free Zone Campaign

What Antoniou and Seralini have found is that GMOs, which are inundated with pesticides like RoundUp Ready containing glyphosate and 2-4-D, the active ingredient in

Agent Orange, create numerous health problems, including birth defects, cancer, neurological imbalances, embryonic deaths, DNA damage, and fetal death.

It's not rocket science to understand that when you eat a steady diet of these horrible chemicals, you will suffer disastrous health ramifications despite the fact that the GMO crops are designed to resist the heavy poisoning of the pesticides and herbicides.

HERE IS EVERYTHING YOU REALLY DID NOT WANT TO KNOW ABOUT GMO FOODS BUT NEED TO KNOW

GMO FACTS by Christina Sarich

GMO foods are not good for our health. There is so much proof in this department; it is insulting that Monsanto would tell us otherwise. The French have proven GMO causes cancer.

http://www.policymic.com/articles/15889/french-gmo-research-finds-monsanto-corn-causes-cancer-america-should-pay-attention.

Other scientific research proves that GMOs cause birth-defects and miscarriage.

http://www.examiner.com/article/mounting-evidence-that-gmo-crops-can-cause-infertility-and-birth-defects

GMO corn has been linked to organ failure.

http://www.huffingtonpost.com/2010/01/12/monsantos-gmo-corn-linked_n_420365.html

The list of genetically modified foods' damaging effects is long, and the evidence is continually mounting against it. GMO even changes our DNA via interference with our micro RNA!

http://naturalsociety.com/genetically-modified-foods/

Now you know why you NEED non-GMO phytonutrient dense Moringa!!!!!!

Russia Bans GMOs

Starting in July, no more GMO products in Russia and all must be labeled. Looks like they beat us to the freedom of information.

Russia will not import GMO products—PM Medvedev
RIA Novosti / Maksim Bogodvid

Russia will not import GMO products, the country's Prime Minister Dmitry Medvedev said, adding that the nation has enough space and resources to produce organic food.

Moscow has no reason to encourage the production of genetically modified products or import them into the country, Medvedev told a congress of deputies from rural settlements on Saturday.

"If the Americans like to eat GMO products, let them eat it then. We don't need to do that; we have enough space and opportunities to produce organic food," he said.

The prime minister said he ordered widespread monitoring of the agricultural sector. He added that despite rather strict restrictions, a certain amount of GMO products and seeds had made it to the Russian market.

Prime Minister Dmitry Medvedev speaks at a meeting of United Russia deputies from Russian rural villages in Volgograd on April 5, 2014. (RIA Novosti / Ekaterina Shtukina)Prime Minister Dmitry Medvedev speaks at a meeting of United Russia deputies from Russian rural villages in Volgograd on April 5, 2014. (RIA Novosti / Ekaterina Shtukina)

Earlier, agriculture minister Nikolay Fyodorov also stated that Russia should remain free of genetically modified products.

At the end of February, the Russian parliament asked the government to impose a temporary ban on all genetically altered products in Russia.

The State Duma's Agriculture Committee supported a ban on the registration and trade of genetically modified organisms. It was suggested that until specialists develop a working system of control over the effects of GMOs on humans and the natural environment, the government should impose a moratorium on the breeding and growth of genetically modified plants, animals, and microorganisms.

Earlier this month, MPs of the parliamentary majority United Russia party, together with the 'For Sovereignty' parliamentary group, suggested an amendment of the existing law On Safety and Quality of Alimentary Products, with a norm set for the maximum allowed content of transgenic and genetically modified components.

There is currently no limitation on the trade or production of GMO-containing food in Russia. However, when the percentage of GMO exceeds 0.9 percent, the producer must label such goods and warn consumers. Last autumn, the government passed a resolution allowing the listing of genetically modified plants in the Unified State Register. The resolution will come into force in July.

So the question to ask is 'what are the other governments waiting for?'

Do GMO foods really affect the birth rate?

I am a little conflicted. The U.S. fertility rate fell to another record low in 2012, with 63.0 births per 1,000 women ages 15 to 44 years old, according to the Centers for Disease Control and Prevention. I always thought that the companies that made condoms had some control. Furthermore, I was certain that the pharmaceutical industry really had a firm grip on the birth control industry. Now the reality is that the GMO industry is the top dog especially when it comes to birth control.

There are many that will deny this, and of course, it may be related to the lack of nutrition in the food. Think about this: "the third generation of hamsters (being fed GMO corn) weren't able to produce babies, so there's real safety issues," says Max Goldberg citing a 2007 paper.

In the image seen here, Irina Ermakova from the Russian Academy of Natural Sciences found that GM soy changed rat's testicles. Not that this should be a surprise since this author has found himself under attack, "Scientists who discover adverse findings from GMOs are regularly attacked, ridiculed, denied funding, and even fired. When Ermakova reported the high infant mortality among GM soy-fed offspring, for example, she appealed to the scientific community to repeat and verify her preliminary results." This was reported by the Institute for Responsible Technology.

Another paper found the same result when mice were fed GMO soy. (Surov et al 2010).[33] Alexey Surov says, "We have no right to use GMOs until we understand the possible adverse effects, not only to ourselves but to future generations as well.

We definitely need fully detailed studies to clarify this. Any type of contamination has to be tested before we consume it, and GMO is just one of them."

It definitely seems to me that if you are aware of a non-GMO nutrient source and you do not make it a part of the protocol, that some of the blame lies with you!

Another Opinion on GMO Foods

We have all heard a great deal about GMO foods, but aside from some papers showing a relationship to GMO foods as potential carcinogens and of course loaded with Roundup, the average person does not know much about them. If you wondered why there are so many allergies, nutritional deficiencies and digestive problems in our society, look at what genetic engineer Dr. Michael Antoniou has to say when interviewed by Jeffrey Smith about Genetic Modification of foods. Dr. Antoniou is on staff at a London University Hospital, and he is a group leader in the Department of Medical and Molecular Genetics with 32 years of experience in genetic engineering technology. This is an excerpt from a seventeen-page interview that basically indicates that whoever is producing GMO foods is rolling the dice and looking to cover up any indications of a GRAS (Generally Recognized As Safe) standard.

Dr. Michael Antoniou—All the biochemistry of the plants is determined by proteins, especially in the form of enzymes. And if you are creating, accidentally, inadvertently truncated proteins, altered structural proteins with different specificity, then you're going to have major changes in the composition - biochemical composition - of that plant. This is where the possibility of creating new allergens particularly can arise, as well as novel toxic substances, because there will be sites by chemical reactions now, perhaps, that were not there before. Small molecules in the plant and dramatic reactions on small molecules that can result in (the creation of) toxic substances as well as benign substances.

Jeffrey Smith: So in other words, if you change the shape of a protein, something that could be harmless and beneficial can all of a sudden be Dr. Jekyll and Mr. Hyde and come out causing damage to the body. Again, I'm assuming, and I know they don't actually check for this stuff before they give them to the market. This whole Zola Proteomics study was done after the corn was released. Alright. Now that we get an understanding of just how irresponsible, I'm using my words, not putting it in your mouth, irresponsible it is to cause all this massive, as I call it, collateral damage in the DNA, possibly increasing the existing levels of toxins or allergens, or introducing new ones, as happened in Mon 810 with the new allergen. So then what kind of tests do they do on animals, and are these competent to discover these types of problems? Can you describe the industry research, which I describe as 'ways to avoid finding problems,' but I want to hear your description because you know what could go wrong when you know what's needed to evaluate to catch it.

Dr. Michael Antoniou: Yes, certainly. This is a very, very crucial point. In the United States, you basically have a deregulated system. So that actually Monsanto—in this occasion they generated them—if they are talking about Mon 810 here, but the other corn and the soy variety, they claim compositional equivalence between the GMO and the non-GMO, except for the one new GM gene, GMO gene, and the product. They're claiming equivalence between the GMO and the non-GMO, and therefore no need for safety evaluation. The FDA, USDA accepts that.

With the current mandate whereby the public does not have to be informed as to whether or not the produce they eat is genetically modified or not, I believe you can take a great deal of comfort in the fact that one of your major nutritional sources is over 30% protein in the form of a non-GMO enzymatically alive plant.

Some of you who utilize moringa for weight management may have noticed plateaus in health changes and weight loss while engaging in a *Moringa oleifera* regimen and when you understand the nature of the changes to the food chain and the increased toxic load to the liver, it will become much more apparent. Toxins all have to be dealt with by the liver. There are only four venues for the body to rid itself of toxins: through the skin, exhaled or in urine or feces.

We are overwhelmed by toxins and pathogens. We are affected by every toxin we ingest, inhale or absorb. Considering the four billion pounds of toxic chemicals dumped into the US environment annually. The liver is already overworked and it is the hardest working organ in the body what happens when the food chain becomes hepatotoxic.

Dr. Michael Antoniou: what Professor Seralini's study found - it is a landmark investigation! First of all, the primary objective of the study was confirmed, in that the signs of liver and kidney damage that we are seeing at 90 days in the Monsanto study did, in fact, escalate into very serious damage, especially in the male animals—because there were female groups and male feeding groups—but especially in the male feeding group. They were dying prematurely from liver and kidney failure.

This is something that peaks during the second year of the life of the animals. So that, in a way, proves the primary objective of the investigation. In addition to that, however, there were a number of important findings. One of the study hypotheses of the study for Professor Seralini was that, actually, any negative health outcome was going to be due to the Roundup. He was not actually expecting any negative health outcome from just feeding the GMO alone without any Roundup application during its cultivation. But actually, he found that the GMO alone, without any Roundup application, was also causing these negative health outcomes, both in terms of kidney and liver damage, but also, quite unexpectedly, in terms of escalating higher tumor incidence.

These facts have been known for some time but the science can be manipulated by using temporal parameters and shortening the length of the study...and we have not even begun to discuss Roundup. When you find people who experience detox reactions shortly after beginning *Moringa oleifera* programs, now you know why. *Moringa oleifera* cannot be found at the level that the Nation receives from that company in Utah anywhere else in the world.

And more on GMO

Why am I continuing to discuss GMO foods? I believe that you need the full impact and today's information will give you some idea as to the pervasive nature of this situation. So now the question you have to be asking is whether or not it was a cover-up by design or serendipity on the part of Monsanto. Another question should be, how did this happen? Endocrine disruption has been linked to consumption of GMO foods. Reported adverse effects of endocrine disruption include declines in populations, increases in cancers, and reduced reproductive function in both sexes. The extent of long-term GMO ingestion suggests that it is dangerous on many fronts. The interview continues with Dr. Michael Antoniou interviewed by Jeffrey Smith about Genetic Modification of foods. Dr. Antoniou is on staff at a London University Hospital, and he is a group leader in the Department of Medical and Molecular Genetics with 32 years of experience in genetic engineering technology and knows what he is talking about.

Jeffrey Smith: So we have these rats (being fed with GMO corn). Now, were there also changes in the hormonal system?

Michael Antoniou: Yes, there were. There were disturbances to sex hormone systems in both the males and the females: testosterone in the males and estrogen in the females. These different test feeds, whether it was Roundup, or GMO, or GMO plus Roundup, seemed to have what we could call an endocrine-disruptive effect. They were disturbing crucial hormonal control systems in the bodies of these animals. And again, just crucially, an important point to bear in mind, all of these negative health outcomes were peaking during the second year of life of these animals. They began to increase during the first year, but they were peaking during the second year of life. This is important, because, in other words, it is long after, way long after, any 90-day feeding study that is currently required by any regulator; and that regulator, at the moment, is only the European Union.

Jeffrey Smith: Didn't the first tumor appear within 30 days after the 90-day mark?

Michael Antoniou: The first tumor appeared actually at four months in males.

Jeffrey Smith: Yes, the fourth month, right.

Michael Antoniou: At the seventh month in the females.

Jeffrey Smith: So, conveniently, right after Monsanto would have closed up shop and said, "These rats are fine." If they had kept it up, one of the rats, the male, may have gotten the tumor and they'd have said, "These rats aren't fine." That's highly convenient there.

Michael Antoniou: It is possible. We need the study to be repeated with a larger amount of animals to really get a clear trend, especially in terms of tumor incidence from these feeds. But as things stand, they are highly indicative of something seriously wrong happening. It would be negligent of any regulator to ignore these findings and dismiss them as somehow flawed. Because if they do, they have to admit that what industry did in the past was also flawed. Professor Seralini did exactly the same experimental design as Monsanto, only extending it and broadening it, which means that if his study design was wrong, then surely Monsanto's study design was wrong. Actually, both were fine. I think as far as what Monsanto did, up to 90 days, was fine. Their mistake was they didn't go longer.

Jeffrey Smith: Alright. You were there on the cutting edge. You were right in the eye of the storm here when this hit on September 19, 2012. This is a really interesting thing. So far, we have shown that the process creates side effects that are not evaluated. You have to evaluate them with animal feeding studies. The industry uses animal feeding studies that are incompetent. We finally come along with an independent study that actually shows that a long-term study is causing massive damage to the rats: early death, organ damage, and multiple massive tumors. What is the result of the scientific community, the press and the regulators to this epic study?

Michael Antoniou: It was quite staggering. Within a couple of hours of the study going public, the scrutiny, it was being dismissed as the experimental design being flawed, and that the outcomes were meaningless. It was being criticized as using the wrong strain of rats, not using or analyzing enough rats, when in fact, Professor Seralini used the same strain of rat as Monsanto. He analyzed the same number of animals as Monsanto. He measured all the parameters that Monsanto did, but only added to them and increased the duration of the study.

Smear and discredit are the usual tactics. If Professor Seralini was really wrong, there would not be an uproar. It would be a small paragraph tucked away in the back section of some newspaper. Instead, the clarion has sounded, and the battle has begun. This appears to be the status quo when a significant economic power takes issue with research findings. GMO foods may, in fact, be truly dangerous.

So by now, you are thinking that you really do not eat much corn and that the risk is not that high...perhaps you have heard of HFCS...high fructose corn syrup. It is in everything and goes by many names on labels: glucose/fructose, iso-glucose, glucose-fructose maize syrup, glucose-fructose syrup, and it is used in soft drinks, baked goods, cereals, processed foods, virtually anything that has been sweetened especially in North America. This has been guaranteed to occur because of the taxes placed on sucrose, particularly foreign sugar, which raises the price of sucrose to levels above most other countries, making HFCS cheapest sweetener.

There are other issues such as the HFCS contribution to obesity (40% of the US population) cardiovascular disease, diabetes (now running amok), and non-alcoholic fatty liver disease. Research suggests that because HFCS is so highly processed that it contributes to weight gain by affecting normal appetite functions.

The Seralini study shows that long-term ingestion of GMO food is causing massive damage to the rats: early death, organ damage, and multiple massive tumors. The bad news is that the Mouse Genome Study, completed in 2002, and the Human Genome Study, completed in 2003 show that mice are 99% genetic matches for humans and thus the testing results (for mice and rats) are applicable. The good news is that at least the food products that are non-GMO are starting to identify themselves since those that are GMO have been relieved of that obligation.

Logic is apparently missing from many aspects of our society. Let us examine some facts and see if we cannot deduce a logical plan of action.

Since the public does not have to be informed about the origin of the foods (GMO or non-GMO) that they are purchasing and consuming **AND** GMO foods have been shown to damage the liver of mice in experimental findings on the safety of GMO foods **AND** Mice have been shown to be a close genetic match for humans and therefore testing has validity **AND** *Moringa oleifera* is hepatoprotective (protects the liver) and experiments using mice have shown that *Moringa oleifera* will repair liver damage **THEN** Logic dictates that since it has become extremely difficult to avoid GMO foods and therefore difficult to avoid liver toxicity and damage, then the obvious protocol would be for everyone to consume *Moringa oleifera*.

Makes sense, doesn't it? Toxins out of the body are always better than toxins inside the body. Obvious the best way would be not to put these foreign substances in but it may take a lot of work as you can see in the next article.

10 Crazy Thing Pesticides Are Doing To Your Body

Agrochemicals, home bug sprays, and lawn treatments could be causing chronic illness in your family.

BY LEAH ZERBE & EMILY MAIN

Pesticides aren't just on the food, the chemicals are inside food, too.

Pesticides are designed to kill, although the mode of action they use to put the stranglehold on pests varies. Whether it's nerve gas—like neurological disruption, the unbalancing of key hormones, or the stunting of a plant's ability to absorb life-sustaining trace minerals from the soil, none of the chemical interventions seems all that appetizing, especially considering that chemical residues routinely wind up on and even *inside* of the food we eat every day. Pesticides are also blamed for diminishing mineral levels in foods.

Agrochemical supporters tend to fall back on a "the dose makes the poison" theory, assuming that small exposures aren't harmful. Increasingly, though, independent scientists are debunking that belief, even proving that incredibly tiny doses could set a person up for health problems later in life. Luckily, eating organic, less processed foods can cut back on your pesticide exposure.

#1 Food Allergies: In one of the strangest links to pesticides to date, researchers from Albert Einstein College of Medicine at Montefiore Medical Center in New York City found an association between food allergies and the levels of a pesticide breakdown product in urine. People with high levels of dichlorophenol, a breakdown product of the herbicide 2,4-D and of chlorine used to disinfect tap water, were more likely to suffer allergies to milk, eggs, seafood, and peanuts. It's not clear what could be happening, says Elina Jerschow, MD, MSc, lead author of the study, but she says it may have something to do with the "hygiene hypothesis." Dichlorophenol acts like an antimicrobial and could interfere with healthy bacterial levels in the gut, which, in turn, could upset the body's natural immune reactions to certain allergens in food.

Prevent it: Go GMO-free. The USDA is about to approve a genetically modified (GMO) corn resistant to 2,4-D, one of the main sources of dichlorophenol in our food supply. If approved, the nonprofit Center for Food Safety estimates that the use of 2,4-D would quadruple, exposing millions more people to potentially food-allergy-inducing pesticide by-products. Buy certified-organic foods and download the <u>True Food Shoppers Guide</u> to avoid nonorganic foods that might contain GMOs.

#2 Memory Loss: Another review from University College London recently concluded that low levels of <u>pesticides</u>, such as those considered safe for farm workers who are exposed on a daily basis, cause significant damage to cognitive function—your memory, the speed at which you process information, and your ability to plan for the long term. The review used data from 14 different studies and looked at organophosphate pesticides, which are some of the most harmful chemicals used in agriculture.

Prevent it: Opt for organic produce. Not only will you be avoiding memory-killing pesticides, but also eating a diet rich in fresh fruits and vegetables will ward off memory loss, according to a study in the *American Journal of Epidemiology*.

#3 Diabetes: Scientists have been noticing a link between pesticides and diabetes for years. The latest evidence comes out of the Endocrine Society's 94th Annual Meeting, where Robert Sargis, MD, Ph.D., released the results of a study that suggests tolyfluanid, a fungicide used on farm crops, creates insulin resistance in fat cells. A 2011 study published in *Diabetes Care* found that overweight people with higher levels of organochlorine pesticides in their bodies also faced a higher risk of developing type 2 diabetes.

Prevent it: To save money on organic fare raised without pesticides, cook with organic dried beans. In the home, avoid using chemical air fresheners and artificially scented products—these things are also blamed for inducing type 2 diabetes.

#4 Cancer: More than 260 studies link pesticides to various cancers, including lymphoma, leukemia, soft tissue sarcoma, and brain, breast, prostate, bone, bladder, thyroid, colon, liver, and lung cancers, among others.

Prevent it: The President's Cancer Panel suggests eating organic and avoiding plastic to lower your risk of environmentally triggered cancers.

#5 Autism & Other Developmental Diseases: How do you get autism? The world's leading autism researchers believe the condition develops from a mix of genes and the pollutants encountered in the mother's womb and early in life. Many insecticides effectively kill bugs by throwing off normal neurological functioning. That same thing appears to be happening in some children. A 2010 Harvard study found that children with organophosphate pesticide breakdown materials in their urine were far more likely to live with ADHD than kids without the trace pesticide residues.

Prevent it: Switching to an organic diet rapidly eliminates pesticide residues in the body.

#6 Obesity: Some agrochemical pesticides act as hormone disruptors, meaning they act like a fake version of a naturally occurring hormone in your body, they block important hormone communication pathways in the body, or they interfere with your body's ability to regulate the healthy release of hormones. More than 50 pesticides are classified as hormone disruptors, and some of them promote metabolic syndrome and obesity as they accumulate in your cells, according to 2012 study appearing in *Environmental Health Perspectives*.

Prevent it: Food isn't the only place where these obesogenic chemicals could be lurking. Avoid canned foods and other foods packaged in plastic. Studies have shown that chemicals, such as BPA and phthalates, in food packaging could play a role in obesity as well.

#7 **Parkinson's Disease:** More than 60 studies show a connection between pesticides and the neurological disease Parkinson's, a condition characterized by uncontrolled trembling. The association is strongest for weed-and bug-killing chemical exposures over a long period of time, meaning it's important to keep these toxic compounds out of your household routine.

Prevent it: Don't turn to chemical interventions to kill bugs in your home or garden. Instead, use natural pest control measures.

#8 **Infertility:** Pesticides spell trouble in the baby-making department, thanks to their bad habit of not staying put. For instance, atrazine, a common chemical weed killer used heavily in the Midwest, on Southern sugar cane farms, and on golf courses, has been detected in tap water. Doctors and scientists point to published evidence tying atrazine to increased miscarriage and infertility rates. Other pesticides cause a plunge in male testosterone levels. A 2006 study found chlorpyrifos, a chemical used in nonorganic apple and sweet pepper farming, and carbaryl, a go-to pesticide in strawberry fields and peach orchards, caused abnormally low testosterone levels.

Prevent it: Avoid the worst summer fruit, the kinds most likely to be laced with toxic pesticides. Instead, choose organic grapes, strawberries, and imported plums.

#9 Birth Defects: Babies conceived during the spring and summer months—a time of year when pesticide use is in full swing—face the highest risk of birth defects. During these months, higher pesticide levels turn up in surface waters, increasing a mother's risk of exposure. Spina bifida, cleft lip, clubfoot, and Down syndrome rates are higher when moms become pregnant during high season for pesticides.

Prevent it: To protect yourself, use a water filter that is certified by NSF International to meet American National Standards Institute Standard 53 for VOC (volatile organic compound) reduction. This will significantly reduce levels of atrazine and other pesticides in your tap water.

#10 Alzheimer's Disease: A recent study published in the journal *JAMA Neurology* found a link between pesticides and Alzheimer's. Researchers specifically found that higher levels of the breakdown product of the nasty insecticide DDT (DDE) in the blood of people seemed to fuel the disease. People with higher levels in their bodies were more likely to be diagnosed with Alzheimer's compared to older people with lower levels. This research by no means uncovered a definitive cause of Alzheimer's, but it's a groundbreaking study that could inspire more research into the possible environmental factors—specifically chemical pesticides—that trigger Alzheimer's, a brain disease that currently affects about 5 million people in the United States.

If the findings pan out through further research, it could mean that testing for DDE levels in the body could lead to earlier diagnosis, which has been shown to help ease symptoms of Alzheimer's.

Prevent It: Eat organic as much as possible. Although banned in the U.S., DDT could still contaminate some imported foods. And to keep your brain strong, exercise regularly and avoid processed foods as much as possible.

Just so you understand the magnitude of the problem, we have reached the stage where xenobiotics, chemicals foreign to the biologic system,[34] are present in the adipose tissue (fat) of 100% of the population.[35] It's not like there is any shortage of potential toxicity with the constant presence of pesticides, food additives, heavy metals, pharmaceuticals, alcohol, tobacco, caffeine and recreational drugs readily available for absorption in our environment even umbilical cord blood of newborns has hundreds of toxic chemicals.[36] Physiological efforts are made to eliminate as many of these chemicals as possible, so they are present in the blood, urine, and feces. When there is an excess, the body stores these unwanted toxins in fat and generally fat deposits remain distal to the most important organs.

So if we examine the finding of the research in the previous article, many of the disorders regularly affecting us (allergies, memory loss, diabetes, cancer autism, obesity, Parkinson's, infertility, birth defects, Alzheimer's) are toxicity related and may be preventable or diminished and certainly *Moringa oleifera* as an organic raw food phytonutrient dense food source make a lot of sense.

CHAPTER 4

Inflammation

'The Long And Winding Road'

"Inflammation is now recognized as an overwhelming burden to the healthcare status of our population and the underlying basis of a significant number of diseases."[37] One of the keys to intervening in the incidence of disease is to look for an effective means of interrupting this process.

If you live long enough, you will have a degenerative condition of at least one of your joints. Omega 3, 6, and 9 fatty acids are found in Moringa oleifera, and the ratio is disproportionately omega 3 fatty acids. One of the most impressive studies that actually links *Moringa oleifera* to derived benefits was the meta-analysis conducted by Goldberg et al. (2007) which will be examined later in this chapter.

Our bodies are equipped with the ability to repair themselves given that the equipment (our organs) have the integrity to function and have not been damaged beyond that point. Inflammation is a major factor in this ongoing problem that leads to a degenerating health status. *Moringa oleifera* definitely intervenes in this process offering the body the ability to heal itself.

As the population ages people have more complaints...Who's listening?

Three decades of seeing patients leave an impact on all doctors and trying to not become inattentive to their complaints on occasion becomes an issue. A common finding is that as a patient's pain gets resolved, their memory of it fades as well and it becomes that they cannot adequately accurately remember it. Enter pain inventories where the patient fills in a pain questionnaire to adequately describe their pain and thus when it is diminished that they will remember how much it hurt. You would be amazed at how many *Moringa oleifera* consumers have noticed this phenomenon and for obvious reasons.

Inflammatory Autoimmune Bowel Disorder Colitis Testimony

My story involving *Moringa oleifera* has to do with how I recovered from an autoimmune inflammatory disorder, Diverticular Associated Segmental Colitis (DASC). At the age of 19, I was diagnosed with Diverticulitis, and I was able to control it by closely watching my diet and avoiding foods that contained small seeds. My grandmother had a colostomy, and my dad had severe diverticulitis, so I knew that there seemed to be a genetic disposition to inflammatory bowel disease in my family.

By the age of 25, dietary management was no longer effective, and the severity caused my doctor to refer me to a gastroenterologist. The colonoscopy revealed that I had DASC and I was prescribed a medication called Asacol (mesalamine) an anti-inflammatory drug specifically for bowel diseases. The standard dosage of Asacol is between two to eight 400 mg. tablets a day. In severe cases, a patient is prescribed twelve a day. My case was so severe that I was prescribed 18 a day.

We were raising four small children, and I was working double or triple shifts, and life was hectic. At times my exacerbation of the attacks would be so severe that I was not able to work my usual job and I had to be assigned to a duty that allowed me not to have any pressure against my stomach as the pain was debilitating. Sometimes I would have to take an antibiotic called Ciprofloxacin 500mg to kill the infection in my colon. This disease was painful, debilitating and could cause me agony at any time. The fact that the medications could no longer control my colitis meant that the next step for me would be surgery.

I did not have surgery and decided to tough it out, and I got to a point where my daily intake of Asacol was reduced to 12 pills a day, which is the dosage for an active severe case of this disease. For more than twenty years, from the early 1990's up until 2012 I was at that dosage. In January 2012, a friend of mine told me that his brother had been using a proprietary *Moringa oleifera* formula to help with Prostate cancer and he suggested that I try it.

I had my first Moringa on February 15th, 2012. The date is etched in my mind…if you had taken the pharmaceuticals that I did for 3/4 of your life, you would clearly recall the life-changing event that eliminated the need for those medications. I initially wasn't crazy about the drink. I didn't like the fact that I had to keep shaking the drink bottle to keep the plant sediment from settling on the bottom of the bottle. The taste was different but not unpleasant.

After drinking the juice for a few weeks, I decided to try to wean myself. I slowly cut back on my daily medication intake. After 8 weeks I was completely off them. I had no pain! In the past, if I had run out of Asacol, within 2-3 days I would be in excruciating pain. Now I was completely off it and had no pain issues, no diarrhea or blood in my stool.

A few months after I started drinking my proprietary Moringa formula, I had a doctor's appointment. When I went into the office, the doctor got his prescription pad out and started writing my prescription. I told him I didn't need anything. This man had been my doctor since 1981, so he immediately questioned what I was talking about. I told him I felt fine, in fact, the best I had felt in years. I then took out a box of my Moringa formula and told him I had been drinking this for about 3 1/2 months, and I didn't need the prescription. He looked skeptical, but knowing my history, listened to me. He told me to stay in touch and let him know if any of my previous symptoms returned.

Several months later my doctor requested I come in and see him. He wanted to know how I was doing. I told him I was great. I said that I had more energy than I had in years. He told me that he wanted me to get a colonoscopy to see what was going on inside my colon. I said that would be great!

On July 23, 2013, I had my scope with my gastroenterologist, and I had my follow-up interview with the GI specialist October 1st. He walked into his office and shook his head. I asked, "what's up doc?" and he smiled. He said "I have never seen such an improvement in anyone. Where you used to have severe disease, there is only slight redness." I showed him the box of Moringa and the Moringa tea that I drink. He told me he knew that this must have been what cleared me up but that he couldn't recommend it to others as it wasn't tested by CFIA (Canada Food Inspection Agency) or Health and Welfare Canada. He actually asked where he could get some for his daughter to try! He then said, "Keep drinking that stuff and I will see you in five years for another check-up."

Moringa changed my life. I had never heard of it prior to January 2012. Up until then, my life involved taking as few as 14 and as many as 20 pills a day. I had to closely watch what foods I ate even a little brown on lettuce leaves would cause me to have a flare-up. No more. Why? MORINGA. I believe MORINGA is a miracle food and I do believe anybody with any type of irritable bowel disease should try it. Why? Because you have nothing to lose and everything to gain. That is WHY MORINGA!

Seizures and MoreTestimonial

About twelve years ago I had to undergo surgery to remove a brain tumor however during that surgery I suffered a stroke. The surgery left me with scarring and nerve damage in my left hemisphere, which impaired my ability to move. I tried every herbal remedy I could find to help with my recovery but had no luck.

Six years later, my fourteen-year marriage ended, and I suddenly found myself a single mother of two, scared and alone. I am not the type of person to let anything keep me down, but despite that mindset, my health was deteriorating. By 2010 I developed Raynaud's phenomenon, a very painful circulation issue, where blood flow to the hands and feet can stop for up to twenty minutes at a time caused by cold or stress, and I certainly had enough stress. I thought I had to deal with this for the rest of my life. If that was not bad enough, in the summer of 2011, I developed seizures, which the doctors thought may be due to the scar tissue from my earlier surgery. I was terrified not only for myself but for my two young children as I was now the sole caregiver.

I desperately hoped for some kind of resolution to my health problems and almost totally missed it. About a month later a good friend of mine talked to me about Moringa oleifera, and although I supported her efforts, I did not do any research on the tree and never tried it.

The next New Year's Eve after celebrating with my friends, ten minutes after I arrived home, I had a seizure. I woke up in the hospital, scared, not knowing what happened. The doctors ran a series of tests and diagnosed me with seizures. They took away my driver's license and put me on meds, telling me that I could get it back after one year with no seizures.

My friend pleaded with me that the Moringa proprietary formula could do a lot for me. I had nothing to lose, so I took it every day, and I started noticing some changes in my health: more energy, wanting to get out of bed, less Raynaud's attacks in my hands and feet. In February I met with the formulator who suggested that I increase my dosage to two servings a day of this proprietary Moringa formula. Three weeks later my Raynaud's attacks stopped. Another three weeks and all my nerves were back! To this day I am seizure free. It works so well for me that I have my two amazing kids that take Moringa every day and they say it wakes them up and makes them think in class. I had been suffering for eleven years, and apparently, all I needed was the Moringa tree.

Omega-3s May Reduce Arthritis Risk

Previous research has revealed a number of studies suggesting that consuming diets containing Omega 3 fatty acids exert a beneficial effect in minimizing arthritis risk. Alicja Wolk, from the Karolinska Institute (Sweden), and colleagues analyzed data collected on a final total of 32,232 women, which involved women born from 1914 to 1948 and living in Sweden during two survey periods, one in 1987 and one in 1997.[38] The first survey contained information regarding diet, height, weight, parity, and education. The second survey expanded the questioning to include smoking history, physical activity, and use of dietary supplements and aspirin. 205 women out of 32,232 women participants developed rheumatoid arthritis during an average of 7.5 years, and 27% of these had Omega 3 less than 0.21 g/day.

After adjusting for confounding factors, women in the highest Omega 3 intake quintile had a 33% lower relative risk of rheumatoid arthritis, as compared with women with lower intake. Analysis of women who completed both surveys (long-term dietary intake) showed that consistent intake of more than 0.21 g/day of dietary Omega 3 was associated with a statistically significant 52% reduction in the risk of rheumatoid arthritis. They found, "Consistent long-term consumption of fish at or more than 1 serving per week compared with less than 1 [serving] was associated with a 29% decrease in risk," the study authors conclude that: "This prospective study of women supports the hypothesis that dietary intake Omega 3 PUFAs may play a role in etiology of [rheumatoid arthritis]."

Now you may want to know why someone who is writing about *Moringa oleifera* is mentioning Omega 3 fatty acids when people commonly associate them with eating fish. *Moringa oleifera* is a wonderful source of Omega 3 fatty acids (it has Omega 6 and Omega 9 FAs also) in perfect balance which means heavily weighted towards Omega 3.

The problem in western diets is that the ratio of Omega 3 to Omega 6 is that it should be 1:2 at the worst since Omega 6 is inflammatory and Omega 3 is anti-inflammatory, but Western diets are yielding a ratio of 1:18 which is highly inflammatory. Since *Moringa oleifera* is plant-based and non-processed, the Omega 3 is absorbed 90-95%, and this potent antioxidant is associated with lengthening telomeres and reducing systemic inflammation.

Arthritis Testimonial

Eight months ago, I received a phone call from an acquaintance, who asked me to google *Moringa oleifera*. She knew about my bad knees (arthritis) and all the different treatments I had tried to alleviate the pain, so she recommended me to try this. At that time, I was extremely distraught because the pain treatments did not work as expected, which meant that I could not work as a sailor. Everything I read made sense, so I started with one pouch daily of the proprietary Moringa formula.

Fortunately, I was not bothered by detox reactions as many people had been, so I increased my dosage a month later, and I was now taking two to three pouches daily. Not long after, I began to notice that the pain in my knees subsided. After nine months absence, being virtually disabled by pain, I could start working at sea again.

I also suffer from Dupuytren's contracture in both hands. This is where the flexor tendons of your hands start to shorten, and you cannot straighten them. I had surgery to try and lengthen the tendons but only on one hand. The other hand had already started to get symptoms of Dupuytren's contracture. Before I started with Moringa, I had trouble straightening the fingers, and there were big hard lumps inside the tendons on my palm. After taking Moringa for about 4-5 months, I suddenly discovered that the hand was improved, and the hard lumps inside the hand began to soften. The lumps are still there, but now it's not so painful and uncomfortable. I am not sure how this plant did this, but I know that *Moringa oleifera* caused my improvement.

Pain & Arthritic Change Testimonial

Growing up I played a lot of (soccer) football and at higher levels as a teen. In my last game when I was 16, I was tackled with such force that I sustained a serious compound fracture of my right knee (patella and tibia). The fracture was so severe that I spent 6 years rehabilitating through physiotherapy, exercise, and massive strength training in order to try to and walk normally, without a limp.

My rehab did not work, and the pain remained so bad that I could only walk up one flight of stairs but never two. If I crouched down into a position where I fully flexed my right knee for more than ten seconds, I had to have someone help me up or use something to hold in order to help myself up. At the age of 40, this is a problem that I have been dealing with for a long time, and it had affected my work because I am the shipping manager at a warehouse that deals in packages between one a hundred pounds and I could not lift or carry these packages.

In addition, about two years ago I lost my warmth after getting sick. Let me explain because only someone who has a fever can understand. I have already felt warm with energy flowing through my body, and my hands were always warm which some people compared to an energy healer. When I got sick, I was freezing even in 30-degree Celsius weather (84 degrees Fahrenheit), and I had to sit around with a blanket, even in that heat with the sun shining on me, just to be warm.

In December 2013 I was introduced to *Moringa oleifera*, and by mid-January 2014 I started taking it, one packet per day. I felt that I had more energy right on the first day. I started to notice changes, so I was interested enough to document them. On the fourth day taking this proprietary Moringa formula, my body heat came back. It was an amazing feeling because I thought that it was gone forever, and I was elated for many days afterward. I felt my knees getting better after about two weeks, and that's when the detox kicked in. I got a pounding headache, and that is when I decided to start taking two packets per day. The headache vanished that same day, and I started losing weight.

My knees continued to improve, and now, five months later, I don't just manage the shipping, I carry a couple of tons a day at work, going just under 8,000 steps each day. I can squat as long as I want, and I get up (without help). I have no problem picking up a 90-pound box off the floor or even running up the stairs...and I have not done this in 25 years. I sleep better and never more than six to seven hours, most often waking myself 5 to 10 minutes before the alarm goes off. In addition, I have also lost 27 pounds (12 kg) since January with no diet.

Decreased Pain Testimonial

I am 31 years old, and I have had three surgeries for prolapsed/herniated inter-vertebral lumbar spine disks. The last surgery was in October 2013. My life was one narcotic painkiller to the next. I was taking up to nine Codeine pills a day but still had pain. I could not empty the dishwasher without having to lie down for an hour on the couch because of severe pain!

Over the last three years, I have tried 10 different painkillers, I but found nothing that could take away my pain and the result without that I was drugged but still in pain. The surgical procedure in October 2013 was successful, but in December 2013 I sneezed, and pain came back making my life hell once again. I was desperate. No one wants to be in pain, and this pain was unbearable. I went with physiotherapist two times a week and continued to medicate myself into a narcotic fog. On January 28, 2014, I decided to stop my physiotherapy to try another course of therapy: working out (training) and conditioning.

The treatment was making my pain worse, and the training made my pain worse. Further, I struggled with joint pain, nerve pain, muscle twitching and spasms, cramps in legs, stomach problems (due to high consumption of drugs) and severe pain in the lower back. That same day I was introduced to Moringa oleifera.

After three weeks of taking a proprietary Moringa formula twice daily, the pain was virtually gone. The twitching and spasms were gone. I was able to sleep at night and had a lot more energy! Now, after 18 weeks on Moringa, I have a new life! I have to say that 3/4 of the pain is gone, and I have more energy, no spasms, much fewer allergies, and my digestive system works! Moringa has changed my life! From day one, I had no blood sugar falls, I sleep better, (awake in the morning) and generally I have more energy! Yesterday I worked for nine hours, and today I am up! My back feels a little fatigued, but two months ago I had been bedridden! The best part of all is that for the most part, I did not hurt anymore! Fantastic!

Osteoarthritis, Inflammation and Heart Disease

So like the bulk of the humans on this planet you are bipedal and therefore subject to the forces of gravity acting on your joints and overtime leading to degeneration and subsequent inflammation. If you have been following my posts, you will understand that there is a definitive relationship between chronic inflammation and chronic disease. Researchers have uncovered another link that will keep you eating your *Moringa oleifera* daily!

Heart Disease Risk Rises with Osteoarthritis

Posted on Dec. 27, 2013, 6 a.m. in Arthritis

Cardio-Vascular Heart Disease Risk Rises with Osteoarthritis Knee Pain

Recently, scientists suggest that inflammation plays a role in osteoarthritis, considered most often to be a disease of "wear and tear." M. Mushfiqur Rahman, from the University of British Columbia (Canada), and colleagues analyzed data collected from 600,000 men and women. The team found that men older than 65 years with osteoarthritis were at 15% increased risk for hospitalization for cardiovascular disease. In addition, women older than 65 years had a 17% increase in cardiovascular risk; women younger than 65 years were 26% increased risk. The study authors submit that: "This prospective longitudinal study suggests that I osteoarthritis] is associated with an increased risk of [cardiovascular disease]."[39]

Do you know a phytonutrient dense plant that has been shown to be a natural cardiotonic and potent anti-inflammatory? Share it with your friends because heart disease is the number one killer.

Many chronic diseases are a result of inflammation. Do you or someone you love have issues because of this?

The literature has been filled with the relationship between inflammation and chronic disease and suggests that as much as 80% of all chronic disease is directly due to inflammation. New research has started to be more specific and give us insight.

Inflammation is the common denominator of many chronic age-related diseases such as arthritis, gout, Alzheimer's, and diabetes. But according to a Yale School of Medicine study, even in the absence of a disease, inflammation can lead to serious loss of function throughout the body, reducing health span—that portion of our lives spent relatively free of serious illness and disability.

Published as the cover article in the October issue of Cell Metabolism, the study found that immune sensor Nlrp3 inflammasome is a common trigger of this inflammation-driven loss of function that manifests itself in insulin-resistance, bone loss, frailty, and cognitive decline in aging.

As the elderly population increases, clinicians are seeing a spike in age-related diseases, but scientists did not fully understand the role of inflammation. What is commonly known is that as we age, our cells change, leading the immune system to produce chronic, low-level inflammation throughout the body. Aging is also a major risk factor for multiple chronic diseases, but according to the researchers, biomedical enterprise spends billions of dollars to tackle each age-dependent disease separately.

"This is the first study to show that inflammation is causally linked to a functional decline in aging," said lead author Vishwa Deep Dixit, professor of comparative medicine and immunobiology at Yale School of Medicine.[40]

The common North American diet is pro-inflammatory by a significant ratio of Omega Fatty Acids alone. Omega 6 is inflammatory and should have a ratio of 2:1 with Omega 3 which is anti-inflammatory. The typical western diet has a ratio of approximately 20:1 which predisposes those of us to chronic disease and increased aging. *Moringa oleifera* with 36 different bioavailable anti-inflammatory phytonutrients (and contains significant Omega 3 fatty acids) makes an excellent choice to combat inflammation based aging and functional decline.

Anti-inflammatory Nutrition

The term **Arthritis** originates from the Greek word for joint (*arthro*), and the ending (itis) meaning inflammation. It is actually an inflammatory joint problem that affects approximately forty million people in the United States alone. Although there are more than 100 different types of arthritis the most common form is a plague to the aging population, osteoarthritis, which is also known as degenerative joint disease.

The other relatively common forms of arthritis are gout (hyperuricemia), pseudogout, rheumatoid arthritis and juvenile idiopathic arthritis. There are pain syndromes like fibromyalgia and autoimmune related arthritis like disorders such as systemic lupus erythematosus, and ankylosing spondylitis, which may involve every part of the body. There is also septic arthritis where an infection actually damages the joint. There are more than one hundred joints in the body and nineteen in each hand alone. With nine carpal bones in the wrist and the continuous use of our hands in daily life, no wonder we have overuse disorders such as carpal tunnel syndrome, tenosynovitis (thumb in video game players), lateral epicondylitis (tennis elbow). Continued overuse with no intervention may result in arthritic conditions later in life.

According to the CDC and based on 2007-2009 data from the National Health Interview Survey (NHIS), an estimated 50 million (22% of adults) have self-reported doctor-diagnosed arthritis. Furthermore 21 million adults (9% of all adults) have arthritis and arthritis-attributable activity limitation.[41] If we further examine the data based on the 2003 National Health Interview Survey, it is projected that 67 million (25%) adults aged 18 years or older will have doctor-diagnosed arthritis in less than twenty years by 2030. An estimated 37% (25 million adults) of those with arthritis will report arthritis-attributable activity limitations by the year 2030.[42]

The consistent symptom is always the major complaint by individuals who have arthritis: joint pain. The pain is often something that the sufferer constantly has and may be located in the affected joint and radiate to the peripheral areas. The pain from arthritis is due to inflammation that occurs around the joint, damage to the joint from the disease, the daily wear and tear of joint (erosion of the joint capsule), muscle strains caused by continued movement through a functional range of motion against stiff, painful damaged joints and of course the subsequent fatigue to the muscles.

Currently, there is no cure for either rheumatoid or osteoarthritis. Treatment options vary depending on the type of arthritis and may include physiotherapy, lifestyle changes (including exercise and weight control), bracing, medications and for those who are aware, natural relief from phytonutrients. We commonly hear about joint replacement surgery for hips and knees as these joints get down to 'bone on bone' a little later in life. Often it is the constant inflammatory condition itself that erodes the cartilage, deranging the joint. If one can decrease the inflammation, the joint damage may be slowed. Medications can help reduce inflammation in the joint which decreases pain and potential future damage but takes a toxic toll on the rest of your body (liver) from the continued ingestion of chemicals.

Many of the clinical studies conducted examining the relationship between nutrition and arthritis have focused on omega-3 fatty acids primarily on rheumatoid arthritis (RA).[43] [44] RA is a chronic, systemic inflammatory autoimmune disease that may affect many tissues and organs, but principally attacks synovial joints causing pain and swelling in the joints.

A number of studies have found that omega-3 fatty acids help reduce symptoms of RA, including, inflammation, joint pain, and morning stiffness.[45] [46] [47] Galarraga et al. (2008) found that people with RA who take n-3 fatty acids were able to lower their dose of non-steroidal anti-inflammatory drugs (NSAIDs), but it does not appear to slow progression of RA, only to treat the symptoms and damage to the synovial membranes of the joint continues.[48]

In light of the progression of RA, decreasing the damage to the synovial membranes will significantly delay the damage. Bahadori et al. (2010) found that oral supplementation of omega-3 fatty acids lengthens the benefits of this therapeutic approach in the treatment of arthritis.[49]

A study by Curtis (2002) indicated that diets rich in omega-3 fatty acids (and low in the inflammatory omega-6 fatty acids) was able to help rebuild cartilage and help people with osteoarthritis (degenerative arthritis). [50] A further study on osteoarthritis (Zainal 2009) found that there were benefits to be derived from increasing intake of omega-3 fatty acids. [51] Omega 3, 6, and 9 fatty acids are found in *Moringa oleifera*, and the ratio is disproportionately omega 3 fatty acids.

One of the most impressive studies that actually links *Moringa oleifera* to derived benefits was the meta-analysis conducted by Goldberg et al. (2007). "The results suggest that omega-3 PUFAs are an attractive adjunctive treatment for joint pain associated with rheumatoid arthritis, inflammatory bowel disease, and dysmenorrhea."[52] Moringa is a rich dietary source of omega-3 PUFAs.[53] [54] When looking at arthritis from a diversity of perspectives, *Moringa oleifera* has been used to treat the pain and inflammatory conditions caused by arthritis, a disorder affecting more than 50,000,000 Americans, and other degenerative diseases. [55] [56] [57] [58] [59] [60] [61]

So you were wondering who might be interested in trying *Moringa oleifera* because it contains thirty-six anti-inflammatories. Most people are aging, and those that do not take care of themselves will face the consequences of poor nutrition. What might happen when they try the most phytonutrient dense plant on the planet that contains a diversity of bio-available natural anti-inflammatory phytonutrients?

LIVER TESTIMONIAL

Now you see it...now you don't

"I visited the doctor for the physical for my life insurance policy, that after a few days I would find out that I had cirrhosis of the liver and hemochromatosis, on top of already taking 4 medications for blood pressure, and one for acid reflux twice a day, and three different vitamins that I was recommended to take. Well, it was more upsetting with this new situation than before because, according to the Doctor, I had very little time left on this earth. You can imagine how I felt; I was not upset because I was going to my home in heaven, but my worry and concern was leaving my son with no parents.

Then I started praying and asking God for a few years to see my son grow and at least reach 18th years old. Praying and crying to the Lord, he sent me a friend that brought me something. She gave me some tea bags and some small sachets with some powder that I did not even know what they were. She said to make this tea and that it would help clean my liver and to drink this sachet in the morning to give me energy, but I just put them on the kitchen counter and left them. In my craziness, I did not put together the fact that I was praying for God to send me something and He had sent me the answer.

A few days later I thought I would try it. So, I started using the tea and the sachets of a proprietary formula of *Moringa oleifera*. In the meantime, I was having lab work every week, and I also had three biopsies of the liver. I was told by the doctor that there was no cure for the blood disease and for my liver condition that they needed more time to research my case.

After 3 or 4 weeks went by, one day the Doctor called me at work and said that he had some news for me. At that moment, I did not want to hear anymore, but the news was that the numbers of the enzymes of the liver had come down a lot and the doctor was surprised. The only thing he said was to continue whatever I was doing, and he wanted to see me the following week. So, when I got home from work every day, the first thing I started doing was making the tea and started drinking more of the Moringa formula that my friend had given me.

Within 8 weeks, my liver was clear; but, with my blood disorder, for which, according to the doctor, there was no cure, he said that the only treatment was to donate blood every so often to improve the blood count. However, within 5 months, all of my labs were good, in fact, they were very good. The Doctor started taking me off of my blood pressure medicine. I also started losing some weight; I was 172 pounds and only 5'2". After just 9 months, I became free from all medications, and I have lost 27 pounds. I feel better now than I ever have in my life!

I got my health back and I got my life back. Now I use the Moringa products regularly. Thank you to Jesus Christ that he sent my friend with the miracle plant products to save my life!"

Your Liver Is The Workhorse Of Your Body

The liver is the workhorse of our bodies and it is bad enough that they have to deal with the four billion pounds (that's right 4,000,000,0000) of toxic chemicals dumped into the North American environment annually and the ten thousand of chemical additives put into our food supply that they do not have to tell you about. Poor choices affect you adversely while good choices are beneficial. So here is the best gift you can give. When your liver is in tip top shape, all physiological functions improve. Here is a small excerpt that may indicate to you what might do this.

Hepatoprotective Activity of *Moringa oleifera* on antitubercular drug-induced liver damage in rats.

Abstract

Oral administration of the extract showed a significant protective action made evident by its effect on the levels of glutamic oxaloacetic transaminase (aspartate aminotransferase), glutamic pyruvic transaminase (alanine aminotransferase), alkaline phosphatase, and bilirubin in the serum; lipids, and lipid peroxidation levels in liver.[62]

The primary function of Moringa oleifera is to repair and protect the liver everything else is simply a side-effect. Give the ones you love *Moringa oleifera* and share the knowledge with everyone you can. Make the good choice! [63] [64]

Allergy and Auto-Immune Testimonial

For the last few months, I have used a proprietary Moringa formula, and I have had some amazing experiences. I am a woman now in my mid-forties. While in my mid-thirties in 2001 I developed a pollen allergy very similar to hay fever but worse. This for some reason progressed in turn and crossed over to include food allergies with worse symptoms than before. The symptoms were so bad, and the common allergy medications did not work.

After continuous doctor visits, it was noted that the allergies, which constantly resulted in hives and swollen blood vessels of the face, had become chronic. I looked grotesque, and this is not something that is good for anyone's self-esteem.

But now, after just over two months using this proprietary Moringa formula, I have managed to cut completely OUT cortisone, and now I only take half as much of the anti-histamine allergy medicines. It is quite incomprehensible. I can even eat and drink quite normally without any major outbreaks.

Also, I struggled with psoriasis on the feet, and it has also been much better. I had two large round sections at the top of each foot, where the skin was dry and white. The itching was terrible. I also had dry skin areas just below the toes itched to the point that sometimes it was unbearable. Now it's mostly gone, and the two major areas on the top of my feet have calmed down. When the dry white skin was peeling off, it looked like I had as two large burns and now they are starting to fade away. It is a pleasure to see how my health problems are slowly disappearing from my life because I had long since given up. I now recommend Moringa strongly recommend to everyone I know who is struggling with health problems. Never give up hope.

CHAPTER 5

Obesity

'Carry That Weight'

Diet and Disease

I have been doing anti-aging research for over 30 years and have advocated the relationship between nutrition and intervention in the disease/aging complex for nearing three decades. This is the primary reason for my choice as a vegetarian, but this path is not as easy to follow successfully as it might seem. There are always the B12, protein, and iron issues but when one adopts an intelligent approach these can be dealt with more than adequately, especially when there is a raw, organic, unadulterated source of *Moringa oleifera* available that is the correct varietal.

Many researchers are finding that strong correlation as well, and the link between diet and disease is now well established. This latest paper indicates that a vegetarian source of nutrition decreases the incidence of disease in women as they enter the middle stages of life.

Convenience and the average western diet are leading us down a path that leads right over a cliff: metabolic syndrome (obesity, inflammation, diabetes and coronary heart disease) and early death. It is not like there is a lack of awareness. Time magazine has devoted numerous covers to the issue. It seems to be more an attitudinal problem and people are accepting it far too easily. Diabetes has become an American epidemic. One of the most available areas for us to intervene and bring this potential crisis to a screeching halt is in serum glucose levels. Let me give to you in a nutshell. Currently, in the US, there are approximately 26.1 million diabetics, and many of them have no idea that they are diabetic.

Best estimates suggest that by 2050 there will be 130 million diabetics which suggests that this problem is out of control to such an extent that they have created a new category: pre-diabetic. There are now nearly eighty million prediabetics in America. This was the solution that was put forth. With no sign of being able to change this downward spiral to diabetes, they merely created a new category. Very recently the estimates have been upgraded in an extremely negative way: by 2020 50% of the US population will be diabetic or prediabetic. They have given up. You have just been handed the ball, and this is a very serious game.

Here are the other statistics. In 1950, 25% of the US population was overweight or obese based on a Body Mass Index (BMI) of 25. By 2010 this number rose to 68% based on a BMI of 30, and this escalated to 70% by 2012 based on a BMI of 32. Out of that 70%, there were 37% who were obese. I am forced to use the past tense because by 2015 the sources in the know indicate that 75% of the population will be overweight or obese and a staggering 41% will be obese. The problem is far worse because most people fail to realize that they have used some legerdemain by raising the BMI indices that were used to define obesity.

Over eighty-five percent of Type 2 Diabetics have virtually created the disease themselves, and we know how to affect it. There is a solution as simple as giving your body the nutrition that it needs in a raw format and breaking the cycle. Moringa oleifera can change the face of health for the nation by affecting serum glucose levels and so many other physiological parameters.

We know that diets do not work. Basically, they are too difficult to maintain and we, for the most part, are not looking at it realistically based on how the physiological integrity is maintained with respect to toxicity. For those of you who have heard me talk about the liver, toxicity, and weight management, you know that your body will not start to break down body fat until; the liver, the foreman of the physiological factory that is you, give it the green light. Fat is a fabulous insulator, and when the liver is overwhelmed by the four toxic exit portals no longer being able to push them out through the lungs, skin, feces or urine, these toxins are stored in fat. Now no matter how dumb we act in regard to putting toxins in (environmental, dietary, etc.), the body is smarter and will try to limit the continuous interaction with the already weakened immune system and insulate them in fat. This leads us to understand that detoxification is the key to weight management.

BETTER MID-LIFE DIET LINKED TO HEALTHY AGING

by Shereen Jegtvig

NEW YORK Thu Nov 7, 2013

(Reuters Health)—The way women eat in their late 50s and early 60s may have some connection to how well they age later on, according to a new study.

Earlier studies examining the benefits of a healthy diet have typically focused on its link to specific diseases or death. The new report took a big-picture view of healthy aging in general. Most health conditions develop slowly over many years. So it's important to look at people's disease risks over the course of their lives—not just in old age, Cecilia Samieri said.

"Midlife exposures are thought to be a particularly relevant period," she told Reuters Health in an email. "For example, atherosclerosis in cardiac diseases (and) brain lesions in dementia, start in midlife."

Samieri is from the Research Center INSERM in Bordeaux, France. She worked on the study with researchers from Brigham and Women's Hospital and the Harvard School of Public Health in Boston.

Their results were published in the Annals of Internal Medicine. The report included 10,670 women who were enrolled in the Nurses' Health Study, a large, long-term study which began in 1976. Women included in the new analysis were in their late 50s and early 60s and had no major chronic diseases in the mid-1980s.

All participants filled out two diet questionnaires, one in 1984 and one in 1986. The researchers assigned women scores based on how closely their diets matched a general healthy eating index or a Mediterranean-style diet.

Next, they followed the participants to see how well they aged through 2000 when women were in their 70s. The researchers defined "healthy aging" as having no major chronic diseases, physical impairment, mental health problems or trouble with thinking and memory.

Compared with usual agers, healthy agers were also less likely to be obese, or smoke and they exercised more in midlife. Fewer had high blood pressure and cholesterol. Women with the highest diet scores were 34 percent to 46 percent more likely to have no chronic diseases or impairment in old age versus those with the worst diets after other health-related factors were taken into account. Although it included only women, Samieri said there is no reason to believe that similar associations shouldn't be observed among both genders.

"We know that a balanced plant-based diet, one similar to the Mediterranean diet, the DASH diet, even MyPlate can be heart healthy," Joan Salge Blake told Reuters Health. She is a spokesperson for the Academy of Nutrition and Dietetics and was not involved in the new study.

Heart disease is the number one killer in America, and being overweight and obese can increase heart risks. "It's never too late to improve on your diet and lifestyle," Salge Blake said.

> Perhaps you know someone that would like to improve their health, have less disease and live longer. If you do not know how to implement this, message me and I will be happy to help.

The Relationship Between Obesity and Disease

The best thing you can do for a child is to not allow them to become obese. This latest paper published in January makes it quite clear about the relationships to disease and you have the tools to affect this. The best thing you can do for anyone who is obese is to offer them your help.

Age-Related Consequences of Childhood Obesity.

Abstract

The severity and frequency of childhood obesity have increased significantly over the past three to four decades. The health effects of the increased body mass index as a child may significantly impact obese youth as they age. However, many of the long-term outcomes of childhood obesity have yet to be studied.

This article examines the currently available longitudinal data evaluating the effects of childhood obesity on adult outcomes. Consequences of obesity include an increased risk of developing the metabolic syndrome, cardiovascular disease, type 2 diabetes and its associated retinal and renal complications, nonalcoholic fatty liver disease, obstructive sleep apnea, polycystic ovarian syndrome, infertility, asthma, orthopedic complications, psychiatric disease, and increased rates of cancer, among others. These disorders can start as early as childhood, and such early onset increases the likelihood of early morbidity and mortality. Being obese as a child also increases the likelihood of being obese as an adult, and obesity in adulthood also leads to obesity-related complications. This review outlines the evidence for childhood obesity as a predictor of adult obesity and obesity-related disorders, thereby emphasizing the importance of early intervention to prevent the onset of obesity in childhood.[65]

If you have any knowledge how to help to combat obesity, you have the responsibility to help someone today. Obesity is plaguing the western world!!!

Increased Body Mass Index (BMI) Significantly Increases Incidence of Type 2 Diabetes and High Blood Pressure

Study results confirm BMI is a direct cause of Type 2 diabetes and high blood pressure

An international team of researchers at the Perelman School of Medicine University of Pennsylvania and Children's Hospital of Philadelphia has found that an increased body mass index (BMI) raised the risk for both type 2 diabetes and higher blood pressure. The results add to mounting evidence about the risks of obesity and are of major importance for the obesity pandemic that is affecting the United States—where two-thirds of adults are overweight or obese—and other countries. According to the findings, published online in The American Journal of Human Genetics, for every 1 kg/m2 increase in BMI—equivalent to a 196-pound, 40-year old man of average height gaining seven pounds—the risk of developing type 2 diabetes increases by 27 percent. The same rise in BMI also increases blood pressure by 0.7 mmHg.

"Our findings provide solid genetic support indicating that a higher body mass index causes a raised risk of type 2 diabetes and high blood pressure," said the study's lead author, Michael V. Holmes, MD, Ph.D., research assistant professor of Surgery in the division of Transplant at Penn Medicine. In the new study, the research team used a recently developed statistical tool called Mendelian randomization (MR), which helps researchers identify genes responsible for particular diseases or conditions (such as obesity), independent of potentially confounding factors such as differences in behavior and lifestyle, which can lead to false-positive associations. In this case, the use of MR virtually rules out the possibility that both a high BMI and type 2 diabetes are caused by a third, unidentified factor. "Whether high BMI raises the risk of adverse outcomes is of critical importance given that BMI is modifiable," said Holmes. "Now that we know high BMI is indeed a direct cause of type 2 diabetes, we can reinforce to patients the importance of maintaining body mass within established benchmarks."

Results of the new study were based on the assessment of the genotypes for over 34,500 patients from previous studies. In addition to the results on diabetes and blood pressure,

Holmes and his colleagues found that an elevated BMI has potentially harmful effects on several blood markers of inflammation. While this could be tied to increased risk for coronary heart disease, the researchers suggest it requires further study.[66]

NEVER BEFORE HAS WEIGHT MANAGEMENT BEEN SO IMPORTANT!

Metabolic Syndrome Gone Testimonial

I am 35 years old, and fortunately, my life has been given back to me. No longer will I fall into the inevitable category of metabolic syndrome and heart disease that has plagued so many that have followed the path of being a college football player. I have a wonderful wife and two great children, and yes, I am a former football player, former history teacher and former football coach. Like many former football linemen, I am a big guy and my weight vaulted to over 415 lbs. when I stopped playing. I had all the issues that come with being that overweight. In late 2009, a close friend, actually one of my former coaches, suggested that he had a product not made from a tree but in fact was the tree that could help me. I began using this proprietary Moringa product and saw immediate improvements in my health: blood sugar, blood pressure (hypertension), and cholesterol all reduced from elevated values to normal values.

I was intrigued by this product because of my poor health and like most people, I did not realize just how poor it was until I saw the changes. Four years after starting my adventure with this remarkable tree, I can say that I have lost more than 100 lbs. the products from this tree have saved my life!

For years I have warned my patients to try not to hurt themselves with what they eat!

For decades now I would say to my patients, "Try not to hurt yourself with what you eat, but try to get your nutrition somewhere." I would receive every conceivable reply ranging from "I don't have the energy to those eating totally organic. The problem still existed that getting their nutrition was a lot of work and most were unable to carry it out leading us to the current state of health: diabetes, cancer, and obesity are ravaging the population. Several authors have tried to bring the public up to speed. "With *Salt Sugar Fat: How the Food Giants Hooked Us*, Pulitzer Prize-winning investigative journalist Michael Moss has laid out the foundation and blueprints of the inevitable future raft of class action lawsuits targeting the food industry for knowingly and scientifically designing products that encourage their over-consumption despite their known and well-understood risks." The food chain is broken, and we have to make our best efforts to separate ourselves from the pack. My interest in Moringa stems from the knowledge that poor nutrition has been linked to the major chronic diseases, immune system dysfunction and premature aging that are affecting the global population leading to a decreased quality of life. *Moringa* delivers nutrition that has systematically been removed from the food chain. Almost eighty years ago the clarion was sounded as evidenced in the following quote," Do you know that most of us today are suffering from certain dangerous diet deficiencies which cannot be remedied until the depleted soils from which our foods come are brought into proper mineral balance?"[67]

Paediatric endocrinologist Dr. Robert Lustig, the author of *Fat Chance: The Bitter Truth About Sugar*, stated that the food industry had sufficient knowledge of the potential harm of their products and still did not react in a positive manner.[68] Investigation has shown that they are targeting the children and foods that were actually advertised as healthy for children, in reality, had higher amounts of sugar per gram than their adult equivalents. According to food industry specialist Julie Mennella, "*What basic research and taste in children is shedding light on—and why the foods that they're making for children are too high in sugar and salt—is they are manipulating or exploiting the biology of the child. I think that anyone who makes a product for a child has to take responsibility because what they are doing is teaching the child the level of sweetness or saltiness the food should be. They're not just providing a source of calories for a child, they're impacting the health of that child*"

In response to the dire situation whereby nutrition has been virtually eliminated from our diets *Moringa oleifera* is the obvious solution. Most commonly authors discuss how the leaves of this extraordinary tree contain seven times the vitamin C found in oranges, seventeen times the calcium in milk, ten times the vitamin A in carrots, nine times the protein of yogurt, twenty-five times the iron in spinach, three times the vitamin E of almonds, and fifteen times the potassium in bananas, but very few ever discuss the relationship to disease.[69]

The real mystery is how this five thousand year-old panacea plant went missing and disappeared from the nutritional horizon. Fortunately it has reappeared. It is the solution to provide nutrition for children. It is the solution to provide nutrition for adults. It is the solution to choosing non-nutritional foods that cause inflammation and obesity.

Hashimoto's Thyroiditis Testimonial

I wanted to share how *Moringa oleifera* has affected my life. Since the age of 21, I have been working around a lot of toxins because I have been a hairdresser for the last 25 years. I have been married for seventeen years, and I have three children. I understand pain and suffering because my mom has Rheumatoid Arthritis and my dad has had seven back surgeries. I have had gestational diabetes with every pregnancy, and it went away all three times. For about 10 years my hands and lower back have been extremely painful. I have gone from doctor to doctor: GP, Osteopath, Anti-aging specialist, Chiropractor, Kinesiologist. I have battled diabetes and my weight since my first pregnancy. After my third child, I developed Hashimoto's Thyroiditis, where my metabolism slowed down significantly, and my list of doctors expanded to include an endocrinologist. Nothing was happening.

I was introduced to *Moringa oleifera* by an old friend of mine, and after I did some research, I decided to try it. Much to my amazement...my hands and lower back stopped hurting instantly! Soon into my new journey, I found I did not crave sugar anymore. I learned that I did not even like it much either. I started losing weight quickly. I had been walking before taking the Moringa to lose weight, but I was so fatigued that I neglected other areas of my life. I never got results or any more energy.

After starting with the proprietary Moringa formula, I can now jog. I can also do exercises that no longer hurt my back, and I am down 40 pounds so far. I have been told by at least ten clients so far that my face looks brighter, and my boss even told me that "I look alive!" I have not felt this good since before my marriage! I just wanted to share my story of how *Moringa oleifera* has truly given me my life back.

Is Diabetes Really Out of Control?

This insight may give you some insight into research. It will also give you the blatant evidence that we are not dealing with conjecture. This is evidence-based science and makes up the bulk of my reading. Convenience and the average western diet are leading us down a path that leads right over a cliff: metabolic syndrome (obesity, inflammation, diabetes and coronary heart disease) and early death.[70] Diabetes has become an American epidemic.

Rest assured that Moringa and metabolic syndrome would be an easy lecture topic to show just how effective this phytonutrient dense plant is to expedite this task. One of the most available areas for us to intervene and bring this potential crisis to a screeching halt is in serum glucose levels. Let me give to you in a nutshell. Currently, in the US, there are approximately 26.1 million diabetics, and many of them have no idea that they are diabetic.[71] Best estimates suggest that by 2050 there will be 130 million diabetics which suggests that this problem is out of control to such an extent that they have created a new category: pre-diabetic. There are now 79 million prediabetics in America. This was the solution that was put forth.

With no sign of being able to change this downward spiral to diabetes, they merely created a new category. They have given up. You have just been handed the ball. Here are the other factors. In 1950, 25% of the US population was overweight or obese which escalated to 70% by 2012. Out of that 70%, there were 37% who were obese. I am forced to use the past tense because by 2015 the sources in the know indicate that 75% of the population will be overweight or obese and a staggering 41% will be obese.

Although linear thinking has labeled this epidemic unstoppable (as indicated by their projections), those who venture outside the box such as Drs. Gabriel Cousens[72], Debbie Drake and I believe otherwise and can prove it. Over eighty-five percent of Type 2 Diabetics have virtually created the disease themselves, and we know how to affect it. There is a solution as simple as giving your body the nutrition that it needs in a raw format and breaking the cycle. *Moringa oleifera* can change the face of health for the nation by affecting serum glucose levels and so many other physiological parameters. [73 74 75 76 77 78 79 80]

Diabetes Type 1 Testimonial

I am a 61-year-old man who was diagnosed with Type 1 diabetes many years ago. I should also mention that I have serious cardiovascular conditions. Over the course of 2008 and 2009, I suffered four diabetic collapses commensurate with related hospital stays. The reason for the collapse was that my blood sugar level plummeted down to zero, which is something Type 2 patients never experience. I was fortunate enough to be in populated areas when I collapsed, and the people around me interacted, and that is perhaps the reason I survived.

When I started taking the proprietary Moringa formula, I received an immediate and dramatic drop in my blood sugar level to such an extent that I had to reduce the insulin doses and, yet my blood sugar levels continued to go down. My insulin needs are still decreasing, and it will be interesting to see at what level will stabilize. Where will this end? Will I have to stop taking insulin? According to medical science that is not possible...but it is clear that this for me is a great balancing act. I wake up at night with very low blood sugar - and I need to get up to get some sugar. The balancing act going on that I want to continue with is normal doses of the proprietary Moringa formula as it has other beneficial physiological effects on the body.

I have found if you have type 1 diabetes, you must be extremely careful when you start with Moringa, especially you must take frequent measurements - more than normal, which is usually just before and after meals or less. When all the above said, this is a road of joy and hope towards better health and a better life overall! So, stand and be brave and active with Moringa. I find that my diabetes also has some special psychological implications such as anger and mild depression which, I must say, has stabilized using the proprietary Moringa formula. Oh, and I should not forget that my cardiovascular issues have improved since I started this regimen, so now I'm looking forward to the next check-up with my doctor.

Something To Think About: Inflammation Is Related to Obesity

Inflammation has been linked as a cause of 80% of chronic disease. You can now count obesity as one of them. The average North American has a diminished amount of Omega 3 fatty acids in their diet and significant amounts of Omega 6 fatty acids. As a matter of fact, the ratio of Omega 3 to Omega 6 should be 1:2 or perhaps even 1:1 for optimal health. It should be noted that Omega 3 has anti-inflammatory properties, and Omega 6 is pro-inflammatory. The current ratio in the North American diet is approximately 1:20 and twenty times the amount of dietary Omega 6 predisposes to inflammation. As you will read below, new findings in a rat study show inflammation is related to obesity (now at almost epidemic proportions in the U.S.), and there is a dietary inflammatory factor with the excess Omega 6.

Obesity is Inflammatory Disease, Rat Study Shows Dec 5, 2013

Australian scientists led by Dr. David Fairlie, have found abnormal amounts of an inflammatory protein called PAR2 in the fat tissues of overweight and obese rats and humans. PAR2 is also increased on the surfaces of human immune cells by common fatty acids in the diet. When PAR2 absorption was inhibited, obese rats on a diet high in sugar and fat researchers found that the inflammation-causing properties of this protein were blocked, as were other effects of the high-fat and high-sugar diet, including obesity itself. Par 2 is a protein sequence is 83% identical to the mouse receptor sequence.[81]

Now when you understand that *Moringa oleifera* contains 36 natural anti-inflammatory phytonutrients and copious amounts of Omega 3, logic dictates that in light of the newly identified relationship between obesity and inflammation, the adoption of a *Moringa oleifera* regimen seems to be the perfect natural intervention.

So Now You Can Too

Is society taking a serious approach to disable disease or is the agenda to disable society? Diabetes is not going away which when we examine the Moringa literature seems ridiculous. How is it that this serum glucose insulin disorder, especially diabetes 2, has become so totally out of control?

Diabetes battle 'being lost' as cases hit record 382 million

By Ben Hirschler

LONDON (Reuters)—The world is losing the battle against diabetes as the number of people estimated to be living with the disease soars to a new record of 382 million this year, medical experts said on Thursday.

"The battle to protect people from diabetes and its disabling, life-threatening complications is being lost," the federation said in the sixth edition of its Diabetes Atlas, noting that deaths from the disease were now running at 5.1 million a year or one every six seconds.

People with diabetes have inadequate blood sugar control, which can lead to a range of dangerous complications, including damage to the eyes, kidneys, and heart. If left untreated, it can result in premature death.

"Year after year, the figures seem to be getting worse," said David Whiting, an epidemiologist and public health specialist at the federation. "All around the world, we are seeing increasing numbers of people developing diabetes."

Just scan the literature below. If the powers that be really wanted to get rid of the problem.... Well you can just come to their own conclusion.

Diabetes, Obesity & Serum Glucose Relationships

Bortolotti M, Levorato M, Lugli A, Mazzero G. Effect of a balanced mixture of dietary fibers on gastric emptying, intestinal transit, and body weight. *Ann Nutr Metab.* 2008; 52;p.221–226.

Cho A S, Jeon S M, Kim M J, Yeo J, Seo K I, Choi M S, Lee M K. Chlorogenic acid exhibits anti-obesity property and improves lipid metabolism in high-fat diet-induced-obese mice. *Food Chem Toxicol.* 2010;48:p.937–943.

Dieye A M, Sarr A, Diop S N, Ndiaye M, Sy G Y, Diarra M, Rajraji Gaffary I, Ndiaye Sy A, Faye B. Medicinal plants and the treatment of diabetes in Senegal: survey with patients. *Fundam Clin Pharmacol.* 2008;22:p.211–216.

Ghiridhari V V A, Malhati D, Geetha K. Anti-diabetic properties of drumstick (*Moringa oleifera*) leaf tablets. *Int J Health Nutr.* 2011;2:p.1–5.

Hossain P, Kawar B, El Nahas M. Obesity and diabetes in the developing world—a growing challenge. I. *N Eng J Med.* 2007;356: p.213–215.

Jaiswal D, Kumar Rai P, Kumar A, Mehta S, Watal G. Effect of *Moringa oleifera* Lam. leaves aqueous extract therapy on hyperglycemic rats. *J Ethnopharmacol.* 2009; 123:p.392–396.

Kaneto H, Katakami N, Kawamori D, Miyatsuka T, Sakamoto K, Matsuoka T A, Matsuhisa M, Yamasaki Y. Involvement of oxidative stress in the pathogenesis of diabetes. *Antioxid Redox Signal.* 2007;9:p.355–366.

Karthikesan K, Pari L, Menon V P. (2010a). Antihyperlipidemic effect of chlorogenic acid and tetrahydrocurcumin in rats subjected to diabetogenic agents. *Chem Biol Interact.* 2010a;188:p.643–650.

Karthikesan K, Pari L, Menon V P. Combined treatment of tetrahydrocurcumin and chlorogenic acid exerts potential antihyperglycemic effect on streptozotocin-nicotinamide-induced diabetic rats. *Gen Physiol Biophys.* 2010b; 29:p.23–30.

Kumari D J. Hypoglycemic effect of *Moringa oleifera* and Azadirachta indica in type-2 diabetes. *Bioscan* 2010; 5:p. 211–214.

Ndong M, Uehara M, Katsumata S, Suzuki K. (2007b). Effects of oral administration of *Moringa oleifera* Lam on glucose tolerance in Goto-Kakizaki and Wistar rats. *J Clin Biochem Nutr*. 2007b;40:p.229–233.

Rana J S, Nieuwdorp M, Jukema J W, Kastelein J J. Cardiovascular metabolic syndrome—an interplay of, obesity, inflammation, diabetes and coronary heart disease. *Diabetes Obes Metab*. 2007; 9:p.218–232

Rivera L, Moron R, Sanchez M, Zarzuelo A, Galisteo M. Quercetin ameliorates metabolic syndrome and improves the inflammatory status in obese Zucker rats. *Obesity* (Silver Spring) 2008;16:p.2081–2087.

Sreelatha S, Padma P R. Antioxidant activity and total phenolic content of *Moringa oleifera* leaves in two stages of maturity. *Plant Foods Hum Nutr*. 2009;64:p.303–311.

Tunnicliffe J M, Eller L K, Reimer R A, Hittel D S, Shearer J. Chlorogenic acid differentially affects postprandial glucose and glucose-dependent insulinotropic polypeptide response in rats. *Appl Physiol Nutr Metab*. 2011;36:p.650–659.

William F, Lakshminarayanan S, Chegu H. Effect of some Indian vegetables on the glucose and insulin response in diabetic subjects. *Int. J Food Sci Nutr*. 1993;44:p.191–196.

If we know about the solution, why don't they?

American Obesity Skyrockets, More Than 50% of Adults are Obese

What Can You Do To Help With The Problem

American waistlines and body fat content are expanding at such a rapid rate that more than half of adults met the diagnostic criterion for obesity by 2009. The prevalence of hyperglycemia (remember yesterday's blog about diabetes) increased by 65%, and one in five of all U.S. adults had elevated fasting serum glucose, according to the *Journal of the American College of Cardiology*. "Evidence of underlying divergent trends in cardiometabolic risk in the adult U.S. population has also revealed an alarming increase in abdominal obesity since 1999, despite apparently stable prevalence of metabolic syndrome during the same time period," Hiram Beltran-Sanchez, PhD, of the Harvard School of Public Health, "Our results demonstrate potential targets for interventions to reduce the future burden of cardiovascular disease (CVD) and type 2 diabetes and confirm the urgent need for multifaceted and coordinated treatment programs to address the increasing prevalence of obesity in the U.S."[82]

"The analysis had two principal objectives: to evaluate prevalence trends for the syndrome and its individual components and to compare time trends in risk factors across racial/ethnic groups and by sex and included 10,814 participants. Subgroup analysis showed variation by racial/ethnic group. Waist circumference increased significantly in whites and blacks but did not change significantly in Mexican Americans, although their rate of abdominal obesity increased from 49.9% to 58.73% over the study period (*P*=0.119)."[83]

The real issue, once you start to look at how obesity affects society and the disease demographic, is that there are strong correlations between this factor and all the major diseases:

cancer, heart disease, and diabetes. The estimates indicate that if there is no intervention in the current trend, the prediction is that a staggering 41% of the US population will be statistically obese by 2015 a major proportion of the 75% that will be overweight or obese by that time.

And If You Are Obese Check Your Heart

If you really want to help someone, here are three reasons to introduce them to *Moringa oleifera*. The first is the fact that *Moringa oleifera* is an adaptogen which attempts to normalize all physiological functions and is very capable.[84] The diversity of phytonutrients in *Moringa oleifera* diminish cravings due to proper nutrition and leptin release leading to weight loss. Excessive weight, independent of all other factors, was just implicated in a significant risk for heart attack and heart disease.[85]

In this very recent paper, heart disease and heart attack which have the highest incidence of all chronic diseases and jockey for first in the fatality list with cancer, are shown to be directly related to a person's weight. Help those who do not know how to help themselves.

You don't have to be a vegetarian... but it helps!

Having been a vegetarian for coming up to thirty years, I cannot remember the taste of meat, chicken or fish. Don't get me wrong, I don't miss it, and they certainly have developed an entire industry surrounding it. That's probably where the problems begin because every industry wants to maximize profit and that's another story about hormones and antibiotics. Before I talk about solutions, let's let the other shoe drop.

Red Meat Consumption and Subsequent Risk of Type 2 Diabetes

"Previously, a number of studies have suggested that red meat consumption associates with an increased risk of type-2 diabetes. An Pan, from the Harvard School of Public Health (Massachusetts, USA), and colleagues explored whether changes in red meat intake affect subsequent diabetes risk. The study included follow-up on 26,357 men enrolled in the Health Professionals Follow-Up study, 48,709 women enrolled in the Nurses' Health Study, and 74,077 women enrolled in the Nurses' Health Study II who reported their diet, including meat derived from mammals, on a food frequency questionnaire every four years. The researchers found that self-reported type 2 diabetes incidence was almost doubled for individuals who moved from low intake of two servings per week up to high intake of seven or more servings per week versus those who stayed at a low level over the 4 years from baseline.

Further, moving from a moderate, two-to-six servings per week, up to high intake boosted risk 87%; whereas shifting from moderate to low intake of red meat lowered risk by 19%. Staying at a moderate intake was associated with 37% higher diabetes onset risk than staying at a low intake. Staying at a high intake was 2.1 times riskier for incident diabetes than staying at a low intake. Cutting red meat consumption to a moderate level had a benefit. The study authors conclude that: "Our results add further evidence that limiting red meat consumption over time confers benefits for [type-2 diabetes] prevention."[86]

Statistics do not lie. The more meat you eat, the higher your risk for type 2 diabetes. If you followed my previous commentary, you realize that there is a nutritional solution to this issue. I commented yesterday on the diabetes crisis and plant-based solution, and I will let you have those references again in a moment. You do not need meat. There is nothing that meat provides that you cannot get from plants. Basically, the public conception is that meat is the best protein source. Meat is 30% anabolic (building) and difficult to digest requiring a great deal of energy.

Soy and whey, which are non-meat based protein sources, are 16% and 17% anabolic respectively but that tree that grows within 700 miles of the equator is 61% anabolic.

If you are worried about strength, gorillas are vegetarian and so are hippopotami. If you are worried about aging, elephants are vegetarian too. All your nutrition is available from plants and plants are more bioavailable, far easier to absorb, and the nutrients have not been mechanically altered by processing. Now with that being said, there is one plant that is head and shoulders above all others, and it is the most phytonutrient dense plant in the world: *Moringa oleifera*.

Steroids are not the only way of enhancing Athletic Performance

Thanks to George Spellwin's article (most of which is below between the lines) to kick off a little comment on athletic performance. Those of you who know me personally realize that this is one of my areas of special interest and we most certainly can achieve tremendous success when we understand the physiology and do not rely on banned substances. The death of Warrior and so many great wrestlers (never assume for a moment that these people are not amazing athletes who suffer a tremendous amount of punishment) should be food for thought and for all those who currently may use these illegal alternatives. George is regarded by many as an expert in the use of steroids.

Steroids in the WWE—Wrestling's Dirty Secrets

After ten professional wrestlers were suspended by the WWE for steroids and the Chris Benoit tragedy, wrestling is in hot water. That's why pro wrestling icons Kevin Nash, Brett Hart, and others appeared on Hannity and Colmes to exchange some heated words in a debate over steroids. Elite Fitness has the exclusive footage right here!

When it comes to professional wrestlers, you normally don't think of them as being very intelligent or articulate. After all, these are the same people who run around a ring hitting each other with steel chairs and sledgehammers while taking breaks in between to throw themselves through tables. And it doesn't help matters that the typical wrestler looks like a sweaty, long-haired, freakishly huge monster.

Karen Hanretty However, if you think that pro wrestlers are just a bunch of crazy, idiotic meatheads, you would be totally wrong and several wrestling legends who recently appeared on Fox News' hit show Hannity and Colmes proved this point as they debated over the issue of steroids in the WWE (World Wrestling Entertainment). One of the wrestlers even convincingly smashed Hannity and Colmes on the subject!

The first interview involved the Ultimate Warrior, or just Warrior as they refer to him now, talking with Sean Hannity. The interview was light-hearted at first, and when Warrior was asked about rampant steroid use in the industry, he said, "Oh, steroids are used throughout the industry all the way through. I mean it's easier to say or point out the number of guys who aren't doing steroids than those that are."

Wrestler Ultimate Warrior Hannity also asked Warrior if he used steroids and he readily admitted that he had used them throughout his career. However, the interview got ugly when Hannity started asking him about roid rage. Before Ultimate Warrior got pissed, he managed to express that, "Roid rage for me is a pie in the sky theory that's thought up by people who have no business discussing the frame of mind of an elite physical athlete."

Warrior started getting louder when Hannity said any use is abuse and insinuated that steroids played a huge role in Chris Benoit killing his family. Alan Colmes then jumped in to calm him down and ask him about why he thinks 60 pro wrestlers under the age of 45 have died in the last 10 years. That's when Warrior gave his best quote of the interview.

He said, "Look, those other guys in the industry, it gets back to the difference between there being use and abuse. Those guys were rotten on the inside (took lots of other drugs besides steroids). I would use this illustration...look at guys like Arnold Schwarzenegger, Frank Zane, Dave Draper, all of the classic bodybuilders. Those guys took steroids, and they're still alive."

There are natural alternatives and athletes who perform at the highest levels and set world records are using these... the safer, smarter choice...we'll miss you Warrior...gone far too soon!

Dementia…it's all in your head

I get asked this question every other day...after I mention mental clarity that is...can *Moringa oleifera* do anything for dementia? You be the judge...it looks good to me!!!!

To date, the preventive strategy against dementia is still critical due to the rapid growth of its prevalence and the limited therapeutic efficacy. Based on the crucial role of oxidative stress in age-related dementia and the antioxidant and nootropic activities of *Moringa oleifera*, the enhancement of spatial memory and neuroprotection of M. oleifera leaves extract in an animal model of age-related dementia was determined. Therefore, our data suggest that M. oleifera leaves extract is the potential cognitive enhancer and neuroprotectant. The possible mechanism might occur partly via the decreased oxidative stress and the enhanced cholinergic function. [87]

http://www.ncbi.nlm.nih.gov/pmc/articles/PMC3884855/figure/fig6/

No wonder mental clarity is one of the hallmarks of those consuming Moringa.

Something to think about...

Moringa In The News

"Moringa's high vitamin A content, almost four times that of carrots, is recognized as a potent micronutrient source to achieve the 2015 millennium development goal to reduce child mortality by two-thirds. Worldwide, an estimated 670,000 children die annually from Vitamin A deficiency."

It should be noted that aside from the fact that carrots used to be considered to be the best food source of Vitamin A, various researchers list *Moringa oleifera* on a gram for gram basis to contain four to ten times more Vitamin A.

Hot off the presses...
Moringa oleifera is exactly what you are looking for!

Review: An exposition of medicinal preponderance of *Moringa oleifera*

Abstract

Medicinal plants are believed to be a precious natural reservoir as they are assumed to have paranormal effects for mankind.

Moringa oleifera grows throughout most of the tropics and has numerous industrial and medicinal uses. This review acquaints with the consequence of fera (Moringaceae), a fast-growing medicinal plant widespread in tropical regions with height ranging from 5-10m. It has an enormous nutritional worth due to the existence of vitamins and proteins. It is subsisted with many constituents. Its oil consists of oleic, tocopherols, stearic, palmitic, behenic and arachidic acid. Flavonoids and phenolics such as gallic acid, chlorogenic acid, ferulic acid, kaempferol, ellagic acid, quercetin, and vanillin are present by means of leaf extract, being richest in phenolics and subsequent fruit and seed extract respectively, that are accountable for antioxidant activity of the plant. Seeds have been pragmatic with active components as novel O-ethyl-4- (α-L-rhamnosyloxy) benzyl carbamate together with seven known compounds, 4 (α-L-rhamnosyloxy)-benzyl isothiocyanate, niazimicin, niazirin, β-sitosterol, glycerol-1-(9-octadecanoate), 3-O- 6-O-oleoyl- β-D-glucopyranosyl-b-sitosterol, and β- sitosterol- 3-X-O -β-D-glucopyranoside, that have been discerned to inhibit EBV-EA (Epstein- Barr virus-early antigen), that is persuaded by the cancer promoter. M. oleifera leaves, gums, roots, flowers as well as kernels have been unanimously utilized for managing tissue tenderness, cardiovascular and liver maladies, normalize blood glucose and cholesterol. It also has profound antimicrobial, hypoglycemic and anti-tubercular activities.

Conclusion

Moringa oleifera has been found to exposit hypolipidaemic, anti-inflammatory, antioxidant, antimicrobial, antifungal, anti-tuberculosis and analgesic effects[88]

Here's the bottom line....Moringa is good for you!

Testimonial...When You're Not Sure of The Diagnosis

I have always been a relatively healthy person. I started competitive swimming when I was 8 years old through the age of 18 and ran track through middle school and part of high school. In college, I typically made homemade meals and after college picked up running again. My whole life I consumed what I considered one of the best supplements on the market.

In May of 2009, when I was 25 years old, I started having difficulty breathing when I ran. However, I just kept training and completed a half-marathon. Symptoms persisted, and the doctor gave me some antibiotics for bronchitis. That didn't work, and my breathing was worsening. The doctor told me that my asthma was flaring up and gave me a steroid inhaler as well as a rescue inhaler. My breathing was so labored that summer that I stopped running and relied on my rescuer inhaler every waking hour. As the summer progressed, I continued to "improve" with the assistance of 2 steroid inhalers and only required the use of my rescue inhaler a couple of times a day.

My third year of teaching began in August of 2009, and the school had a breakout of many sick children and teachers. I was often missing half or ¾ of my class for at least a month. I kept my room as disinfected as possible, kept the windows open, and we washed our hands many times throughout the day. There were very few of us that didn't miss any days of school during that time period, and I was one of them.

In early October, my uncontrollable coughing began. At first, it was just a tickle in my throat so I would lightly cough to alleviate it. My cough kept going until it developed into a major coughing fit. I had to gingerly hold my rib cage with one arm and brace myself with the other arm so I wouldn't fall over. I would have a coughing fit, catch my breath, slowly lift my head from the dizziness, and keep going about my day. The teachers always knew when I was at school because they could hear me throughout the building. I sought out a different doctor, saw him several times, and he kept telling me it was my asthma flaring up and that the allergens were really bad that year. In December, I asked to be referred to a pulmonologist.

The pulmonologist had me do a pulmonary function test, with potentially fractured/bruised ribs from the coughing and took 13 vials of blood. The nurse also did not add the extender to the needle.... The results came back that I had "small airways disease." However, I could not find any information about it. While the diagnosis did not make sense to me, I continued to follow the regime given to me.

In December, I started noticing heaviness in my legs. I assumed I was just tired from the coughing and the side effects from the medications. I struggled to get out of bed in the morning, but the doctors did not seem concerned by my levels of fatigue because of my age. The principal at my school shared his concerns about my health and was very persistent that I should get to the bottom of it. His advocacy for me kept me going when multiple doctors told me "women handle stress differently than men" and prescribed me anti-depressants. I took one of them for a week and got so sick from it that I lost 10 pounds. Against my doctor's orders, I took myself off the medication knowing that I was not stressed or depressed. I just wanted to be healthy and active again!

Finally, around February of 2010, I was given a medication geared towards pertussis that knocked the coughing out of me. I was hoping that I would recover and move forward, but I didn't. My gait and energy levels worsened. At this point, I had to convince myself that I could stand up and put one foot in front of the next.

I kept seeking out different specialists and was prescribed another steroid along with many other medications. One day at school mass, I was barely able to keep my head up and felt disoriented. I got up, walked slowly out of the church, and collapsed. I couldn't walk at all and was taken to the emergency room. They couldn't find anything wrong with me and prescribed me Percocet, Vicodin, and another painkiller even though I clearly stated that I was in no pain. The teachers pitched in and told me to stay home for at least a week and rest. I figured if this is stress related then this is a great opportunity to recover! I had no lesson plans, no grading, and nothing to take care of except for me!

After a week on bed rest and relaxation, I went back to school. I had slightly more energy and was hopeful. However, my walking and overall wellness were still poor. I continued to seek out doctors. My sister-in-law, a physical therapist, observed my gait over the Easter holidays. As a result, she and my mom scheduled an appointment for me at a research hospital in May of 2010. I had one doctor tell me that I was walking poorly because my legs weren't very strong; however, my sister-in-law did a PT exam and told me that I was strong enough to kick her across the room if I wanted. My older brother described me as walking like a 90-year-old arthritic woman, and my younger brother looked at me with fear in his eyes. The doctors at the research hospital ran a range of tests from asthma and allergies to MS and Parkinson's.

Everything was coming back that I was a pillar of health except for my heart rate. Going from sitting to standing, it spiked up to 180 beats per minute! From a short, very slow walk, it would take 10 minutes to return to a resting heart rate. My body was inexplicably working in overdrive. My family knew something was seriously wrong not only because of how I was walking but because my face was ghost white and my eyes were glazed over, sunken in, and had dark circles around them.

Later in May of 2010, I decided that the poke, prod, and prescribe method was not working. I was done hearing "we will have you better in 4-6 weeks." I figured I had some kind of undetectable degenerative disease, and that I would just have to make the best of my life.

Once the school year was over, I decided to leave teaching mostly due to my health issues. It was not fair to the children that I didn't have the energy level necessary to be a quality teacher. I went from being a teacher that would teach English class while we ran around outside and jumping up on desks to being succumbed to a wheelchair on my worst days whispering to my students to come to me to ask their question. I was not even strong enough to project my voice on some days. After teaching all day, I would lay on the couch all evening barely able to grade papers, and my husband would have to gingerly carry me upstairs to go to bed at night. (A year prior I had hiked and climbed Mt. Hyalite in Montana and stairways became my new mountain.)

Around this time, my aunt and uncle called to share a proprietary blend of *Moringa oleifera* with me. I was sure that it wasn't the miracle they deemed it to be. I have a cousin that is a top-ranked doctor, and she told me that it would not hurt me to try it. Within 24 hours of consumption, my heart rate improved by 10 beats per minute. Within 3 days, I had a noticeable improvement in my walking and energy levels. Within a week, I no longer had the "asthma burn" in my chest and did not require the use of my inhalers anymore. (I have only used my rescue inhaler 1 time since May of 2010!) Within 2 weeks, I was jogging. It was fast, but I was doing it without thinking about it! Because I was so excited about feeling better, I set a training goal that day to compete in a half-Ironman the following year.

I continued to improve with only one minor setback. In the summer of 2010, my family and I walked around D.C. on an intensely hot day. I started feeling the heaviness in my legs that day. Once I cooled off, I was fine.

Training for a race that includes 1.2 miles of swimming, 56 miles of biking, and 13.1 miles of running is rather intensive. I felt so powerful having my body back! In January of 2011, I noticed a dry patch of skin by my right ankle. I didn't think anything of it, but it never went away. It got worse in the summer of 2011, but I attributed it to being irritated by my training.

In September of 2011, I completed the Steelhead half-Ironman competition! It was incredible! My body felt strong, and I had minimal lactic acid build up. The last couple of miles, I was passing men much more athletic than me because their bodies were cramping... and mine was not! I finished the race strong, jumping up and down! My recovery was incredible. Sitting in the car for about 6 hours straight after that kind of race would typically result in muscle stiffness and soreness. I kept drinking my *Moringa oleifera*, got out to walk a couple of times, and was moving around great! Two days after the race, I walked around the state fair for eight hours just like I normally would without any muscle soreness, fatigue, or stiffness.

The rash on my leg worsened, and my health started plummeting again. I actually went off of my *Moringa oleifera* for a few weeks, and that is something I will not do again. My asthmatic symptoms started flaring up again, my energy levels dropped dramatically, and my legs started feeling heavy again.

Last time I was combating my health issues I sought out over 10 specialists, but this time around I had world-renowned resources from which to seek counsel. It was time to finally get to the bottom of my health issues especially since I had a very inflamed, painful, seeping, and solid rash from ankle to my knee, my face was swollen, and my energy levels were dropping. After one test, I was finally able to get a diagnosis! I was diagnosed with the following: skin sensation disturbance, edema, chronic malaise and fatigue, multiple chemical sensitivities, slow transit constipation, gastritis/dysfunction, candida/yeast/fungal/mold infection, adrenal insufficiency, IgA immunodeficiency, myalgia and myositis, lumbago/back pain, pathogenic/pathognomonic bacterial infection, multiple parasitical infections, and gluten/gliadin sensitivity/reactivity.

With all of that going on in my body, there is no way I should have been physically capable of training for and completing a half-Ironman! The amazing nutrition, anti-inflammatories, and adaptogenic qualities in *Moringa oleifera* gave my body the fight it required to go from a wheelchair on my worst days to a half-Ironman a little over a year later. With the assistance of an incredible doctor, I was able to rid my body of the health issues that I had been experiencing for years.

As of November 2012, my health is FINALLY back on track and here to stay! The proprietary blend of *Moringa oleifera* will continue to be my supplement of choice as I live my life to the fullest—hiking mountains, snow skiing, water sports, MMA, competing in an Ironman someday, and just living life!

Thyroid Testimonial

At 44 years of age, I should have more energy and be healthy, but instead, I have major problems with my health. I am on a 60% disability pension due to metabolic problems. Initially, I had an overly active thyroid, and I was treated with radioactive iodine to slow it down. Now my thyroid barely works, and I have a slow metabolism and no energy.

I struggle through the day, and after a few hours of physical labor, I feel like someone hit me with a bat. I have to sleep before I can do anything else. I also do not sleep well, and it takes a long time to fall asleep, and then I get up at 4:30 AM, exhausted after too few hours of sleep.

After taking a proprietary *Moringa oleifera* formula in the morning for three days I can do physical labor for 6 hours without sleep afterwards. Now I fall asleep right away and stay asleep until the alarm clock wakes me in the morning. I have more energy, sleep better and longer and I am always in a much better mood.

Hypothyroid Testimonial

At the age of 27, I was diagnosed with hypothyroidism , and I am now 47 years old. Since being diagnosed 20 years ago, my weight kept creeping up until I hit 168 pounds. I started on the *Moringa oleifera* proprietary formula. Now after six months, I have lost 32 lbs. and went from 168 to 136 pounds. I am only 6 lbs. away from my goal. My hypothyroidism symptoms consisted in a lack of energy every day by the mid-afternoon, depression, frequent headaches, joint pain, extreme difficulty losing weight and maintaining any weight loss, swelling in my feet and lower legs (from the calf down), and my sugar levels were on the borderline of diabetes. Taking Moringa has helped me with most of these symptoms .

Before starting the Moringa regimen, I visited two endocrinologists because of my lack of energy and not being able to lose weight despite four months of constantly working out. These specialists had nothing new to tell me and were no help. After attending a seminar about Moringa, I tried the product for a month and instantly noticed a difference. I had energy that lasted me the whole day, and I was starting to lose weight with more ease. I had no problems playing tennis throughout the whole summer, without feeling burnt out and weak. My sugar levels have also come down to the normal values.

For those of you thinking of jumping on the *Moringa oleifera* bandwagon

I like to piece together the human physiological puzzle and reduce it to terms that allow clear choices to be made by those that understand how health really works. We are facing an increasing number of neurodegenerative diseases, and the numbers increase as the population ages. Food chain issues, absolutely but I will not start on that at this time. There has been a great deal of encouraging results in this area from those who have chosen to include *Moringa oleifera* as a whole food portion of their diet. The following paper may yield insight.

ETHNOPHARMACOLOGICAL RELEVANCE:

Abstract

Moringa oleifera Lam. (Moringaceae) by virtue of its high nutritional as well as ethnomedical values has been gaining profound interest both in nutrition and medicinal research. The leaf of this plant is used in Ayurvedic medicine to treat paralysis, nervous debility and other nerve disorders. In addition, research evidence also suggests the nootropic as well as neuroprotective roles of *Moringa oleifera* leaf in animal models. The aim of the present study was to evaluate the effect of *Moringa oleifera* leaf in the primary hippocampal neurons regarding its neurotrophic and neuroprotective properties.

Materials and Methods

The primary culture of embryonic hippocampal neurons was incubated with the ethanol extract of *Moringa oleifera* leaf (MOE). After an indicated time, cultures were either stained directly with a lipophilic dye, DiO, or fixed and immunolabeled to visualize the neuronal morphology. Morphometric analyses for neurite maturation and synaptogenesis were performed using Image J software. Neuronal viability was evaluated using trypan blue exclusion and lactate dehydrogenase assays.

Results:

Moringa oleifera leaf promoted neurite outgrowth in a concentration-dependent manner with an optimal concentration of 30µg/ml. As a very initial effect, MOE significantly promoted the earlier stages of neuronal differentiation. Subsequently, MOE significantly increased the number and length of dendrites, the length of axon, and the number and length of both dendrite and axonal branches, and eventually facilitated synaptogenesis. The β-carotene, one major compound of MOE, promoted neuritogenesis, but the increase was not comparable with the effect of MOE. In addition, MOE supported neuronal survival by protecting neurons from naturally occurring cell death in vitro.

Conclusions

Our findings indicate that *Moringa oleifera* extract promotes axodendritic maturation as well as provides neuroprotection suggesting a promising pharmacological importance of this nutritionally and ethnomedically important plant for the well-being of the nervous system.[89]

These investigative results strongly suggest that there is a high correlation for the empirical findings that we are finding in those who have neurodegenerative or neurological issues.

The Importance of Protein

In today's busy world, optimal nutritional supplementation will not only help you to feel your best but help you to achieve total health. There is a wonderful and complex process that occurs in your body that directly relates to your fitness. Metabolism describes the rate that biochemical processes in the body provide energy for the maintenance of life. Energy can neither be created nor destroyed merely; transformed from one state to another. Think of your body as a nutritional bank. By making sufficient deposits, many transactions may be carried out each day. The importance of dietary protein has been somewhat underestimated by the general population.

Most people understand that muscle and tissue are made up of structural proteins and that DNA is a specific ordering of amino acids, but how many people realize that protein: makes up our antibodies, controls the distribution of water between intracellular and extracellular compartments, transports hormones, provides nutrients and oxygen for tissues, buffers the plasma, and makes up blood clotting factors, enzymes, neurotransmitters and hormones. Individuals with protein deficiencies have weakened immune systems and may be predisposed to a number of diseases.[90] More importantly, the dietary deficiency of protein has a major impact on morbidity and mortality in children and infants suffering from inappropriate feeding habits.[91]

What Are Amino Acids?

Amino acids are composed of carbon, hydrogen, oxygen, nitrogen, and in some cases sulfur. Amino acids are one of the basic nitrogen-containing substances that go into the synthesis of all proteins in living matter. When dietary protein is digested, proteolytic enzymes separate the components (amino acids) and then carried to the liver. The liver manufactures about 80% of these amino acids. However, there are nine essential amino acids that must be received from dietary sources. Amino acids are subsequently sent to tissues where new cells are being created or sites where old damaged cells are being repaired. Amino acids are primarily absorbed in the small intestine, but small peptides (groups of amino acids) are absorbed directly through the cell membranes and recombined into specially manufactured proteins.

In order for your body to function properly, it needs to create over 40,000 specific proteins (*Protein comes from the Greek word "first things."*) from singular amino acids, daily. Your body manufactures a diverse number of proteins that are responsible for a broad range of functions (from bone growth to maintaining healthy biological terrain pH). Hemoglobin is one of these complex proteins, which is responsible for carrying oxygen to all cells. Enzymes are also complex proteins and are necessary for all aspects of metabolism. Amino acids directly govern how the body works and functions.

The nutritional value of protein is determined by its amino acid content. This is why amino acids are called the building blocks of protein. Ingested proteins are hydrolyzed by the digestive system and then combined into the specific proteins needed for growth and to maintain good health.

The quality of any protein is indicated by the essential amino acid content because the ratio of these amino acids will dictate their efficacy in the body for their ability to manufacture the necessary physiological components. If the ratio of essential amino acids is incomplete, the effects will be significantly reduced. Moringa oleifera contains not only the eight essential amino acids but in fact all twenty amino acids utilized by the body.

Net nitrogen utilization is the absolute indicator of the value of any protein. All nutrients ingested can only follow the anabolic or catabolic pathway. The designation associated with the biological value of a protein is the net nitrogen utilization (NNU). The NNU indicates the percentage of a protein that follows the anabolic (building) pathway. Soy, whey and casein proteins range between 14% to 17% anabolic.

What this means is that only 14% to 17% of these proteins will be used for building other proteins and 86% to 83% will follow the catabolic pathway and be digested and disposed of as feces.

The reason protein diets have been effective is due to the fact that they offer the least amounts of nutrient to the catabolic pathway and an individual's body will use stored fats and glycogen to burn for the energy to carry out metabolic functions such as weight loss A chicken egg was previously thought to have the highest NNU value of any protein in the human food chain at 48%, meaning 52% enters the body as calories. When digesting protein through the catabolic pathway, one must be concerned with nitrogen catabolites. A hen egg protein releases 52% nitrogen catabolites, formerly the lowest among any dietary protein until the assays of *Moringa oleifera* came to light. Nitrogen catabolites are considered metabolic, toxic waste, therefore, is recommended in the dietary management of patients with renal or hepatic failure to diminish the dietary content.

When your diet provides essential nutrients but reduced calories, you will lose weight, but more importantly one must examine the nutrition being delivered to your body. Naturally occurring proteins are far more bioavailable than altered, modified, isolated and genetically modified proteins being offered on the market today as supplements. *Moringa oleifera* has, by far, the highest NNU ever provided by any known dietary protein containing 1.3 times the essential amino acids of eggs. Protein quality will determine not only how you appear but how well your body functions. Proteins will control not only the rate but if some physiological actions occur and all of these factors will affect function and health. Most amino acid supplements are the results of some laboratory concocting a formula derived from animal, egg, or yeast protein. Very few are solely plant-based or the plant itself.

Leucine, isoleucine, and valine are the three essential amino acids that make up approximately 1/3 of skeletal muscle in the human body and all present in *Moringa oleifera* and play an important role in protein synthesis, muscle growth, and muscle recuperation after exercise or injury. Many supplements are not absorbed quickly and when bonds have to be broken and naturally occurring plant-based amino acids when used properly can help maximize muscle growth and recovery following intense exercise. By ingesting amino acids whether from food sources or as a supplement, the body does not have to catabolize muscle tissue to derive extra energy. The fact that *Moringa oleifera* is more than 30% protein is the reason that it has been so effective at treating protein malnutrition.

Environmental Chemicals and Health Risks

There are many out there who are driven by agendas that are less than humanitarian...some driven by profit, others driven by ignorance. From my perspective, pointing out glaring dangers that may go unnoticed and offering a solution is the natural philosophical evolution of the altruistic cognoscenti. Those that tear down and challenge for reasons known only to themselves will have to look in the mirror one day. We should all look only to help other people excel because quite frankly nothing else is logical.

According to the annual report of the 2009 President's Cancer Panel, which focused on the link between environmental exposure to chemicals and health risks, there are more than 80,000 synthetic chemicals used in the U.S. Some of the chemicals potentially hazardous to human health—bisphenol-A (BPA), benzene, formaldehyde, and dioxin—have been in the public spotlight recently, but the vast majority are unknown to most consumers. Some of these chemicals are carcinogenic, and with approximately 1.5 million Americans diagnosed with cancer every year and roughly 562,000 Americans dying from various forms of cancer in 2009 alone, it is imperative that consumers are educated to the potential risks of these substances, so they are empowered to act preventively for the sake of human health. These chemicals are largely unregulated and understudied, with only a few hundred being adequately tested for safety. U.S. Department of Health & Human Services, President's Cancer Panel: 2008–2009 Annual Report, Reducing environmental cancer risk: What we can do now?

The best way to detoxify is to consume enzymatically alive, non-processed whole food green plants. Some of the blue-green algae work well also. It does not matter if it is lettuce, chlorella, broccoli or the most phytonutrient dense plant, *Moringa oleifera*. If you want to combat your unavoidable exposure to environmental toxicity choose the one that fits into your demographic. I have made my choice.

While we're on the subject of detoxification…

The largest organ in our body is actually on our body. It is the skin, and there are approximately twenty square feet of skin in the average person. The skin is the organ that is responsible for the absorption of many toxins, and there are about 80,000 different chemicals being dumped into our environment on a regular basis.

Our second largest organ, the liver, is a three-pound dynamo involved in most of the millions of physiological processes in the body and known to carry out more than five hundred functions. Probably the best-known function of the liver is detoxification, but it has many other important roles. There is something that you can do to help your liver out and detox the rest of your body.[92][93][94]

People commonly ask two questions. How soon should I start my child on Moringa? How long will it take to detox? There are billions of pounds of more than 100,000 different toxic chemicals released into the environment annually. Forty-two billion pounds of toxic chemicals either manufactured or imported into the US daily. Everything you ingest, inhale or absorb will be sorted out by your immune system and excreted or stored. The simple answer is that toxins are always better outside of the body. Would you be surprised to know that almost 10 years ago they sampled umbilical cord blood in newborns and found an average of 287 chemicals in each newborn?

Body Burden: The Pollution in Newborns
The Pollution in Newborns
THURSDAY, JULY 14, 2005

A BENCHMARK INVESTIGATION OF INDUSTRIAL CHEMICALS, POLLUTANTS, AND PESTICIDES IN UMBILICAL CORD BLOOD

Environmental Working Group, July 14, 2005

Summary. In the month leading up to a baby›s birth, the umbilical cord pulses with the equivalent of at least 300 quarts of blood each day, pumped back and forth from the nutrient- and oxygen-rich placenta to the rapidly growing child cradled in a sac of amniotic fluid. This cord is a lifeline between mother and baby, bearing nutrients that sustain life and propel growth.

Not long ago, scientists thought that the placenta shielded cord blood—and the developing baby—from most chemicals and pollutants in the environment. But now we know that at this critical time when organs, vessels, membranes, and systems are knit together from single cells to finished form in a span of weeks, the umbilical cord carries not only the building blocks of life, but also a steady stream of industrial chemicals, pollutants and pesticides that cross the placenta as readily as residues from cigarettes and alcohol. This is the human "body burden"—the pollution in people that permeates everyone in the world, including babies in the womb.

In a study spearheaded by the Environmental Working Group (EWG) in collaboration with Commonweal, researchers at two major laboratories found an average of 200 industrial chemicals and pollutants in umbilical cord blood from 10 babies born in August and September of 2004 in U.S. hospitals. Tests revealed a total of 287 chemicals in the group. The umbilical cord blood of these 10 children, collected by Red Cross after the cord was cut, harbored pesticides, consumer product ingredients, and wastes from burning coal, gasoline, and garbage.

This study represents the first reported cord blood tests for 261 of the targeted chemicals and the first reported detections in cord blood for 209 compounds. Among them are eight perfluorochemicals used as stain and oil repellants in fast food packaging, clothes, and textiles—including the Teflon chemical PFOA, recently characterized as a likely human carcinogen by the EPA's Science Advisory Board—dozens of widely used brominated flame retardants and their toxic by-products; and numerous pesticides.

Of the 287 chemicals we detected in umbilical cord blood, we know that 180 cause cancer in humans or animals, 217 are toxic to the brain and nervous system, and 208 cause birth defects or abnormal development in animal tests. The dangers of pre- or post-natal exposure to this complex mixture of carcinogens, developmental toxins and neurotoxins have never been studied.

Thank you to the Environmental Working Group for everything you do! *Moringa oleifera* users know about the powerful detox caused by ingesting *Moringa oleifera*. It is never too early.

Here's Why You may Feel Ill Somewhere Into Your Moringa Protocol

Moringa oleifera, a tree that can grow in the worst climatic conditions and thrive where others cannot, maybe the most phytonutrient inclusive plant on this planet. With somewhat more than one hundred nutrients and countless functions, *Moringa oleifera* can cause the body to combat, mitigate or overcome more than three hundred diseases according to the National Institute of Health.[95] This African/Asian tree is capable of delivering what the body needs and these enzymatically active amino acid sequences may simply not exist in the food chain anywhere else, and that is just the tip of the nutritional iceberg when it comes to *Moringa oleifera*.[96][97][98]

Enzymatically active bio-available *Moringa oleifera* provides thirty-six natural anti-inflammatories, contains forty-six different anti-oxidants, has potent anti-pathogenic properties, and ample amounts of chlorophyll and minerals such as zinc and magnesium.[99][100][101][102] Somewhere into your *Moringa oleifera* regimen pathogens will die, fat will break down releasing stored toxins, and the magnesium, the top metal in the reactivity series and core element of chlorophyll will start to displace the heavy metals stored in your body. The phyto-nutrition in this formulation is so potent that you will feel it almost immediately. Your body will also react to all the negative factors that have been displaced.

Anytime you ingest, inhale or absorb any substance your immune system must deal with it. What you cannot eliminate via urine, feces, sweat or exhalation must be dealt with by your immune system which is clearly looking to sort out self from non-self. Often times toxic chemicals are stored in the fat, usually the omental fat which lies atop your abdominal viscera. Many times microorganisms can hide from our overworked immune system and wreak havoc at some later point in time when our resistance is down, like Lyme disease.

When you begin a regimen that can kill pathogens and chelate or evict heavy metals and other toxins, there are 'detox' reactions. The Jarisch-Herxheimer reaction feels similar to a bacterial infection and can occur after the beginning of antibacterials such as penicillin or tetracycline, or the intervention of a potent anti-pathogenic plant. The same phenomenon may occur when Lyme Disease causing agents or *Candida* are killed, and the toxins from inside the dying microorganisms leak into the body. Characteristically, the death of these microorganisms and the associated release of these endotoxins occurs faster than the body can remove the toxins and may manifest as aches, anxiety, cramps, diarrhea, headaches, fever, flu-like symptoms, flushed skin, chills, decreased blood pressure, fatigue, increased heart rate, joint pain, hyperventilation, inability to sleep, increased urination, mood swings, muscle pain, nausea, pains, rashes, restlessness, sinus pain, skin lesions (boils, hives, etc.), and vasodilation.

Virtually any symptom may occur as the immune system has to identify and react to all these toxic threats. Heavy metals and other chemicals may produce similar results. I personally will never forget the removal of my amalgam fillings and the subsequent two months of mercury toxicity that reduced me to a mere ebb of my usual energetic self.... I must assume the dentist really wasn't quite that holistic. Thank goodness for the subsequent chlorophyll protocol that I initiated. This was before the time that there was any commercially viable organic, raw, unadulterated *Moringa oleifera* that I could trust not to be grass clippings.

The intensity of the reaction indicates the severity of the response to the toxic threat. The reaction commonly occurs within a few hours to a few days of the Moringa regimen but is usually self-limiting in a few days. The allopathic remediation indicates an anti-inflammatory agent to try and stop the progression of the reaction and the fact that *Moringa oleifera* is abounding with anti-inflammatories will accelerate this phase. If at all possible continue with your protocol and you will find that these symptoms will pass quickly and a return to well-being will be hastened and surpassed as you strive for optimal health.

If You Thought You Were Toxic? Testimonial

At the time of writing this, I am a 39-year-old recovering opiate addict, and I have been clean of opiates other than Methadone since March 2012, If you are not familiar with addiction, a Methadone program seems like a government-sponsored get high program, but this truly is not the case if the program is worked. I decided when I entered this program to clean my act up once and for all because I had been struggling with addiction since I was 13. So I went on Methadone, being told time and time again by people at the clinic, "no one comes off methadone."

Today I am now nine days free of methadone... to wean, you must decrease. To decrease, you must suffer withdrawal. The withdrawal is unbearable, sweats, nausea, aching bones inside, constant watering eyes, yawns for no reason for hours at a time, cramping of the feet and hands to the point where you can't make them straight. You are housebound until YOUR body decides it is done torturing you for what you have done to it. We all know where that leads us addicts /junkies:

institutions, death, or another attempt to rehab....and the fear to be suddenly CUT off!

This harsh reality is where my story begins with, what I call MY miracle drink, my body replenisher. I just can't say enough good things. I was weaning my Methadone to the point that the doctor was concerned that I would go into withdrawal and I had started with severe cramping and the almost permanent fetal position warding off the pain. I was looking at my FB, and my friend was raving about this Moringa plant, so I asked for help.

Within a week of starting the proprietary moringa formula, my feet and hands were normal, and there was no more pain when I walked. My achy muscles were not so achy! My withdrawal headaches were far and few between, and I KNOW that was the Moringa formula because last time I went through rehab, I had those headaches for years... This wonderful plant saved me and got me through the majority of my withdrawal. There are some things that are just inevitable no matter what you are drinking when coming off opiates.

Today, I drink my proprietary moringa formula in double doses until I am completely detoxed. Tonight I will use a detox tea to help rid myself of any of the toxins lingering in my system. I am grateful for today and tomorrow because I now get to see it with clearer eyes, a new perspective and a daily drink that offers my body a pile of goodness.

Bags of water.... No much more than that

In the first generation of Star Trek where William Shatner was Captain James T. Kirk, there was an episode where humans were described as being bags of water. While this is partially true since we are at least 70%-75% water, there are some things you might want to know. Humans are merely expressions of protein, a number of different amino acids sorted out by our DNA to create everything. When people think about protein, they usually relate protein and muscles and the fact that athletes seem to require this more than others. They do not consider that enzymes, immunoglobulins, neurotransmitters, blood clotting factors, bone, DNA, RNA, and all tissues have core components of protein. Every function is related to protein. Absorption of nutrition from plants is approximately 90% while absorption from supplements is 10% to 25%. *Moringa oleifera* is more than 30% protein and therefore an extremely effective source of protein nutrition.

One of the important uses of protein is the need to make hormones. *Moringa oleifera* contains copious quantities of zinc, which is essential for over two hundred hormones and regulating the secretion of insulin hormone. As the production of insulin becomes normal, the levels of sugar also remain normal in our bloodstream. Every physiological function in the body is mediated by hormones.

Toxins are always better out of the body

So you may have had the experience of having someone try *Moringa oleifera* and then say within a few days, "I can't take this, it's making me sick." So with the experience, you have had you now realize that this person is going through a 'detox reaction.' The problem now reverts to the philosophy that "I was feeling good before but now I am having all these symptoms."

So you tell them, "It's important to get rid of these toxins so your liver will function better and you can improve your overall health."

They have never heard of this and go out to contribute to the $200 billion dollar fast food industry. You may feel bad that they did not listen, but I would say, There's another person who won't be walking up the big hill on the 18th hole carrying their clubs at 85 years old." All the notes in bold are mine interspersed in this article.

So here's a little ammunition for you. "The French National Institute of Health and Medical Research (INSERM; France) warns that ingested foods may contain low levels of thousands of chemicals; and that these polluted foods, individually and in combination, may wreak havoc with the body's metabolic functioning. *(This is the confirmation, not the speculation).*

Employing a lab animal model, Brigitte Le Magueresse-Battistoni and colleagues fed two groups of mice a high-fat, high-sucrose enriched diet. One group then received a cocktail of pollutants added to its diet at a very low dosage. These pollutants were given to the mice throughout—from pre-conception to adulthood *(Just like everyone on this planet).*

Although the researchers did not observe toxicity or excess of weight gain in the group having received the cocktail of pollutants, they did observe a deterioration of glucose tolerance in females, suggesting a defect in insulin signaling. **(*This is a major observation because people may feel fine and continue their anti-healthy activities)*** Study results suggest that the mixture of pollutants reduced estrogen activity in the liver through enhancing an enzyme in charge of estrogen elimination. In contrast to females, glucose tolerance was not impacted in males exposed to the cocktail of pollutants. However, males did show some changes in liver-related to cholesterol synthesis and transport. *(The liver is the workhorse of the body, and when it does not function optimally any adverse physiological actions occur).*

This study authors warn that: "Because of the very low doses of pollutants used in the mixture, these findings may have strong implications in terms of understanding the potential role of environmental contaminants in food in the development of metabolic diseases."

And this is why you need to go on a course of *Moringa oleifera* for at least 120 days or, like the smart people, for the rest of your life.

And why are people so toxic?

Everything you ingest, inhale or absorb must be sorted out by your immune system or liver, and consequently, your liver is overworked. With only four venues of detoxification (skin, lungs, urinary or fecal) often times your body is unable to dispose of the vast amount of toxins in our environment. Just to let you know how affected we may be by the environmental pollutants look at the quote below and realize that these figures are eight years old. Do you think the numbers are less now?

Michigan Bar Journal September 2010

Americans are bombarded with environmental exposure to chemicals from the time they are in utero until after death, with up to 42 billion pounds of chemicals being produced or imported daily in the United States.... Some of these chemicals are carcinogenic and with approximately 1.5 million Americans being diagnosed with cancer every year and roughly 562,000 people dying from various forms of cancer in 2009 alone, it is imperative that consumers are educated to the potential risks of these substances.[103]

But wait! It gets worse.

Dr. Russell Blaylock - What Chemtrails Are Doing To Your Brain

http://consciouslifenews.com/chemtrails-doing-brain-neurosurgeon-dr-russell-blaylock-reveals-shocking-facts/1160096/

Now considering all the potential sources, that is billions of pounds daily! Now those of you in this Nation may now understand why you are seeing such potent detox reactions from people consuming the *Moringa oleifera*. What you may not realize is that the copious amounts of magnesium in this phytonutrient dense plant will kick out metals such as mercury lead and arsenic. Significant detoxification leads to people experiencing decreased pain, better memory, increased alertness and awareness, better sleep, improved sex drive, improved digestion and blood levels of cholesterol and triglycerides. Keep eating your Moringa!

Moringa is too expensive...

So you say you cannot afford to take Moringa and I say the evidence is overwhelming that you cannot afford to not take it. Mike Adams, The Health Ranger, expressed it perfectly when he said, "You can't put a price tag on being healthy... It's priceless." Remember when reading the following article that extracts and isolated supplements are only absorbed 10% to 25%, and plants are 90% to 95% so just think of how better off the subjects in this study would have been with the most phytonutrient dense plant on the planet.

Dietary Supplements Reduce Hospital Burdens

Posted on Sept. 27, 2013, 6 a.m. in
Healthcare and Information Dietary Supplementation

Stays in a hospital can often be lengthy, and some conditions have a high readmission risk. Tomas Philipson from the

University of Chicago (Illinois, USA), and colleagues analyzed more than 1 million adult inpatient cases in the United States, and found that patients provided oral nutritional supplements during hospitalization benefited from 21%, or 2.3 days, reduction in length of stay; and 21.6%, or $4,734, reduction in patient hospitalization cost. Additionally, there was a 6.7% reduction in the probability of a 30-day readmission in patients who had at least one known subsequent readmission and were provided oral nutritional supplements during the previous hospitalization. Writing that: "Use of [oral nutritional supplements] decreases length of stay, episode cost, and 30-day readmission risk in the inpatient population," the lead author submits that: "Because oral nutritional supplements are formulated to provide advanced nutrition and calories for patients and are relatively inexpensive to provide, the sizeable savings they generate make supplementation a cost-effective therapy."[104]

True Value

When one does not know the value of something, they may tend to ignore or overlook that item. We cannot know everything, but we can know where to find trustworthy information. Now let's make it personal. Suppose you were walking down the street and saw a penny lying on the ground and said to yourself that it was only a penny and your back was achy, so you did not bother to investigate and look more closely at it. You saw Abraham Lincoln's profile and kept walking. How surprised would you have been to hear the person walking behind start screaming with delight as he picked up the 1943 copper alloy penny worth about $2 million?

As a doctor having practiced for decades and given advice to patients who did not listen or who were not compliant…. I have seen many people walk by that 'penny' so many times that I could not count. It used to bother me. You cannot make someone listen although you know the value of an action. *Moringa oleifera* is that 'multi-million dollar penny' in the health arena. The value of retaining one's health and protecting yourself from free radical and inflammatory attacks on your body prevalent in our environment is more valuable than that 'penny.' Give your body what it needs, and your body will make its best effort to restore homeostasis. When I talked mitochondrial aging to patients, it was usually the penny with a sore back syndrome.... if they only knew?[105]

CHAPTER 6
Aging

'When I'm 64'

Aging is controlled by environmental factors and our mother's DNA (and *Moringa oleifera* nicely eliminates the majority of environmental factors)

According to Ross et al. (2013) over the course of aging our cells change and become damaged. Researchers at Karolinska Institute and the Max Planck Institute for Biology of Aging have shown that aging is determined not only by the accumulation of changes during our lifetime (environmental factors) but also by the genes we acquire from our mothers." [106]

There are many causes of aging that are determined by an accumulation of changes that impair the function of bodily organs. Of particular importance in aging, however, seems to be the changes that occur in mitochondria. "The mitochondria contains their own DNA, which changes more than the DNA in the nucleus, and this has a significant impact on the aging process," said Nils-Göran Larsson, Ph.D., professor at the Karolinska Institute and principal investigator at the

Max Planck Institute for Biology of Aging, and leader of the current study.

Lars Olson, Ph.D., professor in the Department of Neuroscience at the Karolinska Institute added, "Many mutations in the mitochondria gradually disable the cell's energy production. This is the first time that researchers have shown that the aging process is influenced not only by the accumulation of mitochondrial DNA damage during a person's lifetime but also by the inherited DNA from their mothers (mDNA). "Surprisingly, we also show that our mother's mitochondrial DNA seems to influence our own aging," said Larsson. "If we inherit mDNA with mutations from our mother, we age more quickly.... Our findings can shed more light on the aging process and prove that the mitochondria play a key part in aging; they also show that it's important to reduce the number of mutations," said Larsson.

(If you have heard me lecture on the role and functions of antioxidants, you know they play a major role in protecting against cellular mutation and cellular integrity by protecting hydrogen bonds).

"These findings also suggest that therapeutic interventions that target mitochondrial function may influence the time course of aging," said Barry Hoffer, M.D., Ph.D., a co-author of the study from the Department of Neurosurgery at University Hospitals Case Medical Center and Case Western Reserve University School of Medicine. "There are various dietary manipulations and drugs that can up-regulate mitochondrial function and/or reduce mitochondrial toxicity. An example would be antioxidants."

We have seen the amazing beneficial effects *Moringa oleifera* has on mice in many of the studies I have cited here and also in my books. Antioxidants protect mitochondria from free radical damage (Reactive Oxygen Species), and there are forty-six of them in *Moringa oleifera*. Aside from environmental factors, mitochondria in their function of creating ATP also create free radicals to damage themselves (Chen et al. 2003).[107] Categorically all the findings in this paper suggesting therapeutic interventions and dietary manipulations are accomplished by the phytonutrients found in *Moringa oleifera* and in particular mitochondrial protection.

USC Announces: Delaying aging is a better investment than cancer, heart disease

news.usc.edu - December 22, 2013 6:58 AM

Even modest success in slowing aging would increase the number of non-disabled older adults by five percent every year from 2030 to 2060

"On the heels of an announcement from Google that the company's next startup, Calico, will tackle the science of aging, a new study shows that research to delay aging and the infirmities of old age would have better population health and economic returns than advances in individual fatal diseases such as cancer or heart disease.

With even modest gains in our scientific understanding of how to slow the aging process, an additional 5 percent of adults over the age of 65 would be healthy rather than disabled every year from 2030 to 2060, reveals the forthcoming study in the October issue of Health Affairs.

Put another way, an investment in delayed aging would mean 11.7 million more healthy adults over the age of 65 in 2060. The analysis, from top scientists at USC, Harvard, Columbia, the University of Illinois at Chicago and other institutions, assumes research investment leading to a 1.25 percent reduction in the likelihood of age-related diseases. In contrast to treatments for fatal diseases, slowing aging would have no health returns initially, but would have significant benefits over the long term.

In the United States, the number of people aged 65 and over is expected to more than double in the next 50 years, from 43 million in 2010 to 106 million in 2060. About 28 percent of the current population over 65 is disabled.

"In the last half-century, major life expectancy gains were driven by finding ways to reduce mortality from fatal diseases," said lead author Dana Goldman, Leonard D. Schaeffer Director's Chair at the USC Schaeffer Center for Health Policy and Economics. "But now disabled life expectancy is rising faster than total life expectancy, leaving the number of years that one can expect to live in good health unchanged or diminished. If we can age more slowly, we can delay the onset and progression of many disabling diseases simultaneously."

The study shows significantly lower and declining returns for continuing the current research "disease model," which seeks to treat fatal diseases independently, rather than tackling the shared, underlying cause of frailty and disability: aging itself."

How does this reflect upon those who know what real nutrition can do for you? I cannot think of a better vehicle to delay the onset of aging than the two-fold approach of reducing chronic inflammation and the protection of telomerase and telomeres. Chronic inflammation may, in fact, be responsible for up to eighty percent of all chronic disease including cell line senescence, which is the death of a cell line where no further replication is possible. Telomeric shortening is aging by definition.[108][109]

Anti-oxidants are able not only to protect telomerase but in fact, Omega 3 fatty acids have been shown not only to reduce telomere shortening but to increase telomere length [110][111], and these are provided in copious amounts by *Moringa oleifera*. Providing proper nutrition increases immune system function and decreases the incidence of disease. When nutrition is provided by fruit and vegetable sources, the outcome is life extension. When natural anti-inflammatory phyto-nutrition is ingested regularly pain from many degenerative diseases diminishes to the point of virtual elimination. *Moringa oleifera* can provide the nutrition necessary to delay aging, decrease inflammation and allow the body to combat disease and therefore places it at the forefront to slow the onset of disease and significantly delay the onset of aging.

Telomere length is also linked to and likely regulated by, exposure to inflammatory cytokines and oxidative stress[112][113][114] and the anti-oxidant, anti-inflammatory profile of *Moringa oleifera* makes it a primary intervention to prevent telomeric shortening.

Give the body what it needs and you will find that the body will press the reset button.

Protect Your Telomeres

SORTING IT OUT AND LIVING LONGER

So what does it all mean? Why have I been letting you know all the problems without a clear solution? I am not going to leave you hanging because the role of every health care practitioner should be to bring about wellness in the least invasive manner with the most efficacious vehicle. For decades I have advised my patients to try not to hurt yourself with what you eat but get your nutrition from a safe source. A very close friend of mine kept on telling me that the people did not understand why I would put up a slide of a man eating a light bulb. She said to remove the slide because it did not get a response and I told her that most people harm themselves with what they put in their mouth and certainly the statistics on disease bear this out. Humans are supposed to be able to survive on air, fluids, and food and food is letting down the bulk of the population. The US Army used to have a great motto,

"Be all you can be" and now we see that there is an inherent danger in GMO food and perhaps that food source will not allow people to be all they can be. No one is giving you the facts.they cut their experiments short so they can say that they didn't find anything. Get your nutrition from a safe source...raw, organic, vegan, enzymatically-alive nutrient rich and try to minimize the foods that damage you. The body is resilient.

Moringa oleifera and telomeres: The Science

"Telomeres are composed of a six-protein telomere-specific complex termed shelterin. The shelterin complex comprises the physical ends of chromosomes and serves to prevent chromosomal ends from being recognized as DNA double-strand breaks (DSBs). The synthesis and maintenance of telomeres are mediated by telomerase, a specialized ribonucleoprotein complex. In the absence of telomerase, the failure of DNA polymerase to fully synthesize terminal ends of the lagging DNA strand leads to progressive telomere shortening with each round of cellular replication. In human tissues, the strict down-regulation of telomerase accounts for the age-dependent decline in telomere lengths in somatic cells. Studies have documented a decrease in telomere length in several human epithelial cell types. This rate of telomere length attrition would be significant in long-lived organisms such as humans leading to cell line senescence. Shortened telomeres are also a consistent finding with the diseases that are the highest incidence causes of death; cardiovascular disease, cancer, and diabetes."

Antioxidants, outside of the carotenoids, enter the electron cascade, which means their combined effect is more than the sum of the effect of the single components. Antioxidants such as vitamins A, C, E, Omega 3 Fatty acids and selenium (all present in *Moringa oleifera*) will release an electron to a free radical and bind it, transforming it into a relatively harmless molecule fit for excretion. Omega 3 fatty acids themselves will not only protect telomeres but have actually been shown to lengthen them. The trace elements zinc and selenium are essential for our antioxidant enzyme system. *Moringa oleifera* contains ample amounts of forty-six bioavailable enzymatically active different antioxidants including Vitamin A and the carotenoids.

A proprietary formula containing assorted parts of the *Moringa oleifera* tree (leaf, leaf puree, fruit, fruit puree and seed cake) ensures a diverse assortment of bioavailable antioxidants. If you want to protect your ability to reproduce existing cell lines, it is critical to protect your chromosomes. If a multivitamin containing extracted antioxidants is able to afford protection for telomere length, the diversity of bioavailable enzymatically active readily absorbable plant-based antioxidants found in *Moringa oleifera* will confer a far more potent protective effect.

I always have been a proponent that our lifestyle choices can move us from the chronological clock to a physiological clock. Professor Helena Baranova corroborated that with her findings that 85%-96% of disease is due to environmental factors. Now another group working under the guidance of the 2009 Nobel Prize winner for her work with telomeres and telomerase, Elizabeth Blackburn, shows us that we can indeed impact the length of our life and our health status. "Telomeres typically shorten during normal cell divisions and, therefore, telomere length and rate of shortening are indicators of mitotic cell age. Telomere shortening is counteracted by the cellular enzyme telomerase. In human beings, telomere shortening is a potential prognostic marker for disease risk and progression and for premature death."

In this paper, the effects of comprehensive lifestyle changes (plant-based diet, moderate exercise, stress management, and increased social support) on telomerase activity in men with low-risk prostate cancer are investigated. After 3 months of intervention, telomerase activity was significantly increased in peripheral blood mononuclear cells.

"Telomere shortness in human beings is a prognostic marker of aging, disease, and premature morbidity. We previously found an association between 3 months of comprehensive lifestyle changes and increased telomerase activity in human immune-system cells. We followed up participants to investigate long-term effects. In conclusion, our comprehensive lifestyle intervention was associated with significant increases in relative telomere length in men with early-stage prostate cancer, compared with active surveillance alone. Adherence to these healthy behaviors was also associated with increased relative telomere length when all study participants were assessed together." [115]

Moringa oleifera is complete plant-based nutrition with hundreds of documented physiological functions. The impressive array of antioxidants in *Moringa oleifera* protects telomerase. This paper may give us some insights as to the bigger picture. By getting involved with a like-minded group involved with sharing the knowledge of this plant would most likely accommodate social support and decreased stress. All you have to do to fulfill the parameters of this study is to eat *Moringa oleifera*, walk every day, perhaps meditate or some other form method to decrease stress (cortisol) and talk with friends. Longer telomeres, longer lives.

Here are more references that show that all physiological indications about the telomeric changes are demonstrated scientific findings and for those that do not believe that Moringa is, in fact, doing what you see with your own eyes... let them follow up the research.

De Lange T. Shelterin: the protein complex that shapes and safeguards human telomeres. *Genes Dev* 2005; 19:p.2100-2110.

Greider C W. Telomeres; Telomerase and Senescence. *Bioessays* 1990; 12:p.363-369.

Harley C B, Kim N W, Prowse K R, Weinrich S L, Hirsch K S, West M D, Bacchetti S, Hirte H W, Counter C M, Greider C W, et al. Telomerase, cell immortality, and cancer. *Cold Spring Harb Symp Quant Biol.* 1994; 59:p.307-315.

Harley C B. Telomere loss: mitotic clock or genetic time bomb? *Mutat Res* 1991;256:p.271-282.

Harley C B, Vaziri H, Counter C M, Allsopp R C: The telomere hypothesis of cellular aging. *Exp Gerontol* 1992; 27: p.375-382.

Lansdorp P M. Telomeres and disease. Review. EMBO J. 2009; 28:p. 2532-2540.

Rodier F, Kim S H, Nijjar T, et al. Cancer and aging: the importance of telomeres in genome maintenance. *Int J Biochem Cell Biol.* 2005; 37: p.977–990.

Hahn W C. Role of telomeres and telomerase in the pathogenesis of human cancer. *J Clin Oncol* 2003;21: 2034-2043.

Kumar N A, Pari I. Antioxidant action of *Moringa oleifera* Lam (drumstick) against antitubercular drug-induced lipid peroxidation in rats. *J Medicinal Foods.* 2003; 6(3): p.255-259.

Bharali R, Tabassum J, Azad M R H. Chemomodulatory effect of *Moringa oleifera*, Lam, on hepatic carcinogen-metabolizing enzymes, antioxidant parameters and skin papillomagenesis in mice. *Asian Pacific Journal of Cancer Prevention* 2003; 4: p.131-139.

Njoku O U, Adikwu M U. Investigation on some physico-chemical antioxidant and toxicological properties of *Moringa oleifera* seed oil. *Acta Pharmaceutica Zagreb.* 1997;47(4): p.87-290.

Siddhuraju P, Becker K. Antioxidant properties of various solvent extracts of total phenolic constituents from three different agroclimatic origins of drumstick tree (*Moringa oleifera* Lam.) leaves. *Journal of Agricultural and Food Chemistry.* 2003;51:p.2144-2155.

Xu Q. Parks C G. DeRoo L A. Cawthon R M. Sandler D P, Chen H. Multivitamin use and telomere length in women. *Am J Clin Nutr* 2009: 89(6):p.1857-1863.

Turning Back The Clock...Testimonial

As I pass through middle-age I have accepted the continual losses of getting old bit by bit: decreasing energy, stiff joints, sore feet, and the list goes on. Moringa changed all that; it turned these annoyances around. After a few months of taking a proprietary moringa oleifera formula the soreness from working out is now minimal or non-existent. The stiffness, due to inflammation has disappeared. Mental clarity has replaced the early morning fog, and pure, clean energy brings me back to how I felt many years ago.

I feel like the clock has been turned back. I haven't had anything dramatic occur as some people have experienced: but the effects of the Moringa have made me feel better, younger, healthier and made me a believer, a life-long user.

The word is getting out

Awareness of Moringa puts you very much ahead of the curve and indicates that you have knowledge of the most phytonutrient dense plant on the planet. Others are starting to hear about it, but you know where to get the most efficacious version of Moringa-oleifera.

Moringa: The Ideal Food for Everybody?

Saturday, 08 February 2014 22:08

PRLog (Press Release) - Feb. 8, 2014 - BERLIN, Germany - The Moringa story must be told as many people are still in the dark about this wonderful blessing from nature. With a world grappling from malnutrition, our hope lies in this plant whose leaves are capable of wiping every aspect of malnutrition out of the world not to talk of the many benefits derived from other parts of it, namely: the seeds, flowers, roots, and bark. Among all the plants I know I cannot think of a more nutritious one than Moringa.

Moringa oleifera—one of nature's best-kept health and nutrition secrets. What is Moringa? For centuries, people in Asia and Africa have had access to *Moringa oleifera*, one of nature's most nutritious foods. Often called the Tree of Life or Mother's Best Friend, it provides families—infants, children, parents, and grandparents—with an abundance of minerals, vitamins, calcium, proteins, and beneficial antioxidants and amino acids. This generous and bountiful plant is life sustaining.

In the world of nutrition and natural health, there are some foods that come out of nowhere and then BAM—one day it's all you hear about. One of those foods is Moringa, often referred to as the Miracle Tree. But unlike some of the hyped up trend-foods of years past, there really are some benefits worth noting when it comes to this one. Without further ado, here are some of the many unknown moringa benefits.

Praised for its medicinal value and ability to purify the body while boosting energy levels, *Moringa oleifera*, is native to the Himalayas of India. Currently, it's growth is most prevalent in Africa, Central and South America, and Asia. But it's effects are being felt around the world and if you are willing to dig a bit deeper, there is evidence that this plant has the potential to kill bacteria and parasites, fight diabetes, lower blood pressure, and reduce inflammation throughout the body.

The word is getting out. Embrace it.

Mowing someone else's lawn?

I have to love it when others trolling the market with adulterated, modified, isolated, nutrient sources try to compete with raw organic plant-based nutrition...so here's what just came across my desk...from my previous posting you know the best most available source of Omega 3. It reminds me of the scene from Crocodile Dundee when the mugger pulls a knife on him, and he says, "Now that's not a knife. This is a knife." *Moringa oleifera* is 'that knife' in the nutrient world...nothing has more phytonutrients and when you can get it in an enzymatically alive format, even better.

Do You Want to Boost your IQ, Mental Clarity, and Attitude?

What if we told you that certain foods and supplements could actually increase your IQ and help your brain function more optimally? It's true! And we've got the studies to prove it.

Feeling Tired, Forgetful or Depressed? Did you know that your brain is made up of 60% fat? Your brain needs the right fats to thrive! It is well known that omega-3 essential fatty acids (EFAs) may contribute to the maintenance of healthy mental function. Symptoms of omega-3 deficiency include fatigue, poor memory, mood swings, and depression, to name a few.

If you find yourself trudging through your day, forgetting what you walked into the room for, or just feeling down, the answer could be as simple as getting adequate omega-3s. Omega-3 deficiency is incredibly common. This is because your body does not produce them on its own—they must be obtained through diet.

Research Proves What Omega-3s Can Do For You

One study concluded that supplementation with the omega-3 known as docosahexaenoic acid (DHA) "improved memory and the response time of memory in healthy, young adults whose habitual diets were low in DHA." Another study found that fish oil exerted "exert positive effects on brain functions in healthy older adults."

"DHA supplementation improved both memory and reaction time in healthy young adults: a randomized controlled trial." American Journal of Clinical Nutrition, May 2013.

DHA supplementation improved both memory and reaction time in healthy young adults: a randomized controlled trial

The group that sent out the email was selling a fish oil product but as I have stated before *Moringa oleifera* is an excellent source of Omega 3 fatty acids with far greater absorption than most other forms. "Docosahexaenoic acid (DHA) is important for brain function, and its status is dependent on dietary intakes. Therefore, individuals who consume diets low in omega-3 (n–3) polyunsaturated fatty acids may cognitively benefit from DHA supplementation. Sex and apolipoprotein E genotype (*APOE*) affect cognition and may modulate the response to DHA supplementation."[116] [117]

So Underated, Absent and Needed... Omega 3 Fatty Acids

A recent study from Harvard University and the Center for Disease Control found that Omega-3 deficiencies cause 96,000 deaths per year. Researchers are finding a copious number of health relationships not only between Omega 3 deficiencies but also benefits and protective effects provided by a moderate intake of this fatty acid. Also, telomere length, which is considered to be a definitive measure of physiological age is effected, and the lengthening of telomeres in immune system cells was more prevalent in people who substantially improved the ratio of omega-3s to other fatty acids in their diet.

Fatty Acids Could Aid Cancer Prevention and Treatment

Aug. 1, 2013—Omega3- fatty acids, contained in oily fish such as salmon and trout, (Editor's note: let's not overlook an extremely abundant plant source *Moringa oleifera*) selectively inhibit growth and induce cell death in early and late-stage oral and skin cancers, according to new research from scientists at Queen Mary, University of London.[118]

In vitro tests showed omega-3 fatty acids induced cell death in malignant and pre-malignant cells at doses which did not affect normal cells, suggesting they have the potential to be used in both the treatment and prevention of certain skin and oral cancers. Omega-3 polyunsaturated fatty acids cannot be made by humans in large quantities, and so we must acquire them from our diet. The scientists were studying a particular type of cancer called squamous-cell carcinoma (SCC). Squamous cells are the main part of the outermost layers of the skin, and SCC is one of the major forms of skin cancer. However, squamous cells also occur in the lining of the digestive tract, lungs, and other areas of the body. Oral squamous cell carcinomas (OSCC) are the sixth most common cancer worldwide and are difficult and very expensive to treat.

Professor Kenneth Parkinson, Head of the Oral Cancer Research Group at Queen Mary's Institute of Dentistry, said: "We found that the omega-3 fatty acid selectively inhibited the growth of the malignant and pre-malignant cells at doses which did not affect the normal cells. While previous research has linked omega-3 fatty acids with the prevention of a number of cancers, there has been very little work done on oral cancers or normal cells. Dr. Nikolakopoulou said: "As the doses needed to kill the cancer cells do not affect normal cells, especially with one particular fatty acid we used called Eicosapentaenoic acid (EPA), there is potential for using omega-3 fatty acids in the prevention and treatment of skin and oral cancers. It may be that those at an increased risk of such cancers—or their recurrence—could benefit from increased omega-3 fatty acids. Moreover, as the skin and oral cancers are often easily accessible, there is the potential to deliver targeted doses locally via aerosols or gels. However further research is needed to define the appropriate therapeutic doses."

Now you may want to know why I am revisiting Omega 3 fatty acids again and the answer is that they keep recurring in the literature. *Moringa oleifera* is a readily bioavailable source of Omega 3 fatty acids and in a format that is far easier to absorb. *Moringa oleifera* is a wonderful source of Omega 3 fatty acids (it has Omega 6 and Omega 9 FAs also) in perfect balance which means heavily weighted towards Omega 3. The problem in western diets is that the ratio of Omega 3 to Omega 6 is that it should be 1:2 at the worst since Omega 6 is inflammatory and Omega 3 is anti-inflammatory, but Western diets are yielding a ratio of 1:18 which is highly inflammatory.

Since *Moringa oleifera* is plant-based and non-processed, the Omega 3 is absorbed 90-95%, and this potent antioxidant is associated with lengthening telomeres and reducing systemic inflammation. You may want to consider putting Moringa oil topically on your skin...topical Omega 3 with antioxidants, anti-inflammatories, amino acids, vitamins and minerals and into your body when you see the diversity of the overwhelming impact on potential interventions that plant-based Omega 3 can have on your health.

There is a great deal of documentation on Omega 3 in Moringa in copious quantity. Moyo (2011) found that dried *Moringa oleifera* leaves contain Omega 3, 6, and 9 FAs and 44.57% of the total fatty acids were Omega 3 fatty acids.[119][120][121]

So here is the real impact. *Moringa oleifera* is a tremendous source of bioavailable Omega 3 Fatty Acid and here is what the research shows that it is related to. When you have difficulty in explaining to anyone, layperson or professional alike, this should be enough to make them re-consider the plausibility.

According to the the University of Maryland Medical Center, "Omega-3 fatty acids are considered essential fatty acids: They are necessary for human health, but the body can't make them—you have to get them through food. Omega-3 fatty acids can be found in fish, such as salmon, tuna, and halibut, other seafood including algae and krill, some plants, and nut oils. Also known as polyunsaturated fatty acids (PUFAs), omega-3 fatty acids play a crucial role in brain function, as well as normal growth and development. They have also become popular because they may reduce the risk of heart disease." The public has yet to realize what an important source of Omega 3 Fatty acid can be found in this nutrient-dense plant.

ADD [122][123][124][125][126][127][128]

Asthma [129][130]

Bipolar – Depression – Psychiatric [131] [132] [133] [134] [135] [136]

Menopause [137]

Cancer Prostate, Breast, Colon, Skin [138] [139] [140] [141] [142] [143] [144]

Alzheimer's Disease -Cognitive Function [145] [146] [147] [148]

Diabetes [149]

Heart Disease [150] [151] [152] [153] [154] [155] [156] [157] [158] [159] [160] [161] [162] [163] [164] [165] [166] [167] [168] [169]

Inflammatory Bowel Disease [170] [171] [172] [173]

Macular Degeneration [174] [175] [176]

Schizophrenia [177] [178]

Rheumatoid Arthritis [179] [180] [181] [182] [183]

Skin [184]

Stress Relief [185]

Vision [186]

General [187] [188] [189] [190] [191] [192] [193] [194] [195] [196]

So here we go again where *Moringa oleifera* can provide nutrition not easily found in the average diet. *Moringa oleifera* is a rich source of bio-available, easily absorbed Omega-3 fatty acid. Omega 3 FAs have a plethora of functions and here is another. For those with metabolic syndrome, (central obesity, hypertension, and deranged glucose-insulin metabolism) ingestion of omega-3 fatty-acids significantly improves cardiovascular function (blood flow and arterial stiffness). In North America where obesity seems to be running rampant, this newly published research reinforces the need for this nutrient in our diets.

Omega 3 FAS Counteract Metabolic Syndrome

Abstract

Metabolic syndrome (MetS) is associated with adverse cardiovascular events and impaired vascular function. In this study, we evaluated the effects of omega-3 polyunsaturated fatty acids (PUFAs) supplementation on vascular function, inflammatory and fibrinolytic process in subjects with MetS. We studied the effect of a 12 weeks oral treatment with 2 g/day of omega-3 PUFAs in 29 (15 male) subjects (mean age 44 ± 12 years) with MetS on three occasions (day0: baseline, day 28 and day 84).

The study was carried out on two separate arms (PUFAs and placebo), according to a randomized, placebo-controlled, double-blind, cross-over design. The diagnosis of MetS was based on the guidelines of Adult Treatment Panel III definition. Endothelial function was evaluated by flow-mediated dilation (FMD) of the brachial artery. Carotid-femoral pulse wave velocity (PWV) was measured as an index of aortic stiffness.

Results

Treatment with PUFAs resulted in a significant improvement from day 0 to 28 and 84 in FMD and PWV ($p < 0.001$ for all). Nevertheless, treatment with placebo resulted in no significant changes in FMD ($p = 0.63$) and PWV ($p = 0.17$). Moreover, PUFAs treatment, compared to placebo, decreased IL-6 levels (p = 0.03) and increased PAI-1 levels (p = 0.03). Finally, treatment with PUFAs resulted in a significant decrease in fasting triglyceride levels from day 0 to 28 and 84 (p < 0.001) and in serum total cholesterol levels (p < 0.001).

Conclusions

In subjects with MetS, treatment with omega-3 PUFAs improved endothelial function and arterial stiffness with a parallel anti-inflammatory effect.[197]

Once again the bottom line is easy. Eat your moringa because aside from the anti-inflammatory effect of omega 3 FAs...there are 35 other anti-inflammatory phytonutrients.!

And another article...

Besides being a good source of protein, vitamins, oils, fatty acids, micro-macro minerals elements and various phenolics, it is also reported as anti-inflammatory, antimicrobial, antioxidant, anticancer, cardiovascular, hepatoprotective, anti-ulcer, diuretic, antiurolithiatic, and antihelmintic. Its multiple pharmaceutical effects are capitalized as therapeutic remedy for various diseases in traditional medicinal system. Further research on this charismatic healer may lead to the development of novel agents for various diseases.

Help Humanity Excel

Today is the day to espouse the thoughts that have created my desire to help humanity excel. This is the day before departing to a conference, and all who attend will reach multiple peaks ranging from the metaphysical to the pragmatic. My thoughts are filled with the diversity of the many idioms relating to the compliance of people for any number of things to such an extent that the study of statistics and trends has become totally integrated to all aspects of life.

The two extremes from the philosophical perspective seem to be 'you can lead a horse to water, but you can't make him drink' and 'when the student is ready, the teacher will come.' So what happens to the horse when the teacher walks by unnoticed? This is the essence of what most people in marketing cannot comprehend. The reality is that the horse will live a shorter less productive life. There is no arrogance in this statement because every 'horse' is allowed to make up their own mind. Free will was the Creator's gift to mankind separating us from the Angels.

For the first twenty years of practice, I was trying to save everyone, whether they wanted to be saved or not. I assumed that health was a gift, not a choice. I started to follow the statistics as they related to health, disease, compliance and tried to determine why logic is absent in so many people. If your goal is to help other people excel, you cannot succeed if they are unwilling to listen or comply. Your enlightenment is not based on your success rate but your intentions and effort.

For years I would hammer on cigarette smokers. Smoking is so illogical, yet the threat of 4000 different chemicals, 200 poisons, and 43 carcinogens in every puff does not dissuade smokers from progressing to their imminent lung cancer. The only reason all smokers do not die from lung cancer is that some die from heart disease first.

Now the teacher in me is frustrated at people not listening, but as a doctor, I realized that everyone has their own agenda and since they have free will can participate in choosing their length of time on this planet. Cigarette smokers still do not have the right to infringe on your health, however, and since second-hand smoke is the third leading cause of lung cancer that is precisely what they are doing (of course cigarette smoking is the leading cause of lung cancer). Your liver has enough to do. Dealing with the toxins from someone else's smoke is somewhat unfair and disgusting.

Environmental toxins accumulate in our tissues especially when the immune system cannot handle the current load, and the liver function becomes less efficient and unable to carry out many of the needed physiological functions successfully. When liver function is affected by the increasing amount of toxins in our bloodstream, we may be affected by storing the excess in fat to insulate the toxins safely, or experience detoxification symptoms such as the following: headaches, skin rashes, fatigue, constipation, flatulence, bloated feelings, exacerbated allergic reactions, and hormonal dysfunction as the body desperately seeks homeostasis.

> **"Whenever I found out anything remarkable, I have thought it my duty to put my discovery on paper, so that all ingenious people might be informed thereof."**
>
> Antoine van Leeuwenhoek

So the moral of these ramblings is to try to help those who will listen and protect yourself and your loved ones first and stay away from smokers. Share don't push.

All Systems Go Testimonial

I was always trying to be healthy, and although I did not consider myself to be suffering from anything, in particular, a friend suggested that I look into Moringa oleifera. I started taking this proprietary Moringa formula once a day in June 2013. I didn´t expect anything really as because I didn´t see myself as ill but I thought it could provide nutrition and I had been concerned about what was really in our food, and I knew that good nutrition could affect how you age. What I have experienced since then is simply unbelievable, and then I went up to 2 daily, and now take 4 every day.

I used to have a bunch of little issues that I had become so used to that it had become routine or accepted and therefore, I just considered it normal. I used to have an itchy scalp for years and just take an anti-histamine pill. If I ever forgot my allergy pill, it would drive me crazy and sometimes lead to more typical allergy symptoms: sneezing and congested nose. Two months on this Moringa and all symptoms stopped so I stopped my meds.

I guess I never realized that I had a sleeping problem because I had been taking sleeping aids for seventeen years. I could not sleep without them. After the third month of taking Moringa, I was able to sleep without any medication. Also, I have lost 20 pounds in 6 months without any effort; it has just fallen away. Before I was constantly hungry & ate huge portions. Now I have to remember to eat....

With noticing these changes, I started to look at other things. These are the things that perhaps people just assume is normal for them. My first hair appointment after starting this Moringa product, the hairdresser said I had a lot of new hair growing out all over the scalp. I didn't even know my hair had thinned as I entered middle age but now my hair is thicker, my nails too. My nails have always broken off before they could start to grow; now I have strong nails that I have to file.

I used to rest several hours a day (in the middle of the day) for several years. I thought it was normal for people to nap in the afternoon but now I wake daily at around 7.30 AM and keep going all day until I go to bed somewhere around midnight.

I have struggled for years with feelings of depression & anxiety, particularly during the winter months and maybe it was because I live in a climate that has winter, but I´d have periods where I would worry and be unhappy for no reason. Since taking Moringa, I do not have these feelings anymore. Now I wonder if most people suffer from all these 'little things' because they certainly would fare much better with this Moringa proprietary formula.

Fourth National Report on Human Exposure to Environmental Chemicals

Updated Tables, September 2013

"The Fourth National Report on Human Exposure to Environmental Chemicals, Updated Tables, September 2013 provides nationally representative biomonitoring data that has become available since the publication of the Fourth National Report on Human Exposure to Environmental Chemicals, 2009. The Updated Tables, September 2013 includes all the updates previously provided in Updated Tables, July 2010 through Updated Tables, March 2013. The Updated Tables, September 2013 present data for 91 chemicals measured in serum pooled samples that have not been reported in any previous Updated Tables. Since publication of the Fourth Report, 2009, 201 chemicals have updated tables and 49 chemicals have been added, for a total of 250 chemicals presented in these Updated Tables."

Face it! If you're not detoxing, you're toxic.

Telomeres and the Truth About Aging

Here's an interesting article from Melanie Haiken on age determination using a new technique but acknowledging telomeres and we know how to influence those.

A team of scientists from UCLA has discovered a new biological clock with the potential to measure the age of human tissue. While preliminary, the research has fascinating implications for anti-aging—if it holds up in further testing. Steve Horvath, a professor of human genetics at the David Geffen School of Medicine at UCLA and of biostatistics at the UCLA Fielding School of Public Health used methylation, a natural process by which DNA is altered over time, to develop an "epigenetic clock" that analyze the effects of age on tissue. In a study published in the October 21st issue of Genome Biology, Horvath and his team found that women's breast tissue ages faster than the rest of their bodies and that cancerous tissue is on average 36 years older than other tissue.

So far, the epigenetic clock is simply a statistical model, and it's much too early to say whether it actually works, says Darryl Shibata, M.D., professor of pathology at the University of Southern California's Keck School of Medicine, who has reviewed Horvath's work.

That said, Shibata believes that a test that could determine the biological age of human tissue would have wide-ranging uses. "Right now, as a human, all you have is your birth certificate to tell you how old you are," says Shibata. But as we've all observed in our daily lives, chronological age doesn't necessarily correlate with biological age. "You can go to a high school class reunion and see that in action," Shibata says laughing.

This isn't the first biological clock scientists have used to measure the aging process. For the past 20 years, researchers have been looking at the length of telomeres—the "caps" on the ends of chromosomes—as a measure of biological age, and researchers have been working towards developing an age prediction test based on telomere length. But that's still in the future, and the research hasn't yet had practical applications in terms of turning back the clock. Horvath's research is also a long way away from usability, but it points us in an exciting new direction.

The UCLA study published today suggests the possibility "that we could compare the ages of different tissues and organs in the same individual," Horvath says, with implications for disease diagnosis and treatment. "If we see a drastic acceleration in tissue aging, that would suggest we should start looking for clues to an underlying problem."

In addition, Horvath and his colleagues analyzed the biological age of "induced pluripotent" stem cells, which are adult stem cells used in research that have been reprogrammed to a semi embryonic state, and found that the cells now have a biological age of zero. Says Horvath: "It provides proof of concept that one can reset the biological clock."

Shibata concurs, seeing applications in future research of anti-aging treatments. "If you had a marker of aging that was reliable, you could use it to study aging itself and anti-aging interventions much more effectively."

As an example, Shibata cites the widely studied theory that calorie restriction can slow the aging process. If we could measure the age of subjects' tissue before and after a trial of calorie restriction, we could find out if it has an effect. "If the answer is no, we'd be saving people a lot of misery," he says laughing. "There are hundreds of things that are thought to possibly slow down aging, and if we had a marker, we could test them. Imagine the trouble we could save ourselves and how much faster we could figure out what works and what doesn't."

http://www.forbes.com/sites/melaniehaiken/2013/10/21/scientists-discover-new-biological-clock-that-measures-aging/2/

Winter's Coming

As they say in 'Game of Thrones,' "Winter's coming," which means to those of us in healthcare translates as SAD is coming. When my golf clubs head into the house for the winter that means only one thing, blues skies will not be smiling at me for the next few months. Somewhere around January-February, we may not see much of the sun in northern climates, and that is when depression strikes in the form of the seasonal affective disorder...SAD. It is believed that people are adversely affected by the decreasing amounts of sunlight and the colder temperatures as the fall and winter progress. This is probably a relationship between Vitamin D, which aids in absorption of all nutrients and the physiological implications leading to the symptoms: depression, fatigue, irritability, difficulty concentrating, decreased sex drive, poor sleep, decreased activity level, increased pain, and carbohydrate craving.

There is a further relationship between B vitamins and carbohydrate craving. Once the sunlight is gone, it is more important that we optimize our nutrient intake and furthermore, there is a relationship between depression and niacin, vitamin B3.

If we delve a little deeper into the relationship between depression and nutrition, we find that niacin has been recommended in conjunction with antioxidants like vitamin C, E beta-carotene, and selenium. That is correct for those of you who have caught on already. Look at the nutrient profile describe in this list: antioxidants. Now many of you may have wondered why you have seen some of the things you have with *Moringa oleifera* and the evidence is quite clear. These are the antioxidants in *Moringa oleifera*:

Alanine, Alpha-Carotene, Arginine, Beta-Carotene, Beta-sitosterol, Caffeoylquinic Acid, Campesterol, Ca-

rotenoids, Chlorophyll, Cholesterol, Chromium, Delta 5-Avenasterol, Glutathione, Histidine, Indole Acetic Acid, Indoleacetonitrile, Kaempferol, Lutein, Methionine, Myristic Acid, Palmitic Acid, Prolamine, Proline, Quercitin, Rutin, Selenium, Superoxide Dismutase, Threonine, Tryptophan, A, B Choline, B1 Thiamin, B2 Riboflavin, B3 Niacin. B6 Pyroxidine, C Ascorbic Acid, E Alpha Tocopherol, E Delta Tocopherol, E Gamma Tocopherol, K, Xanthins, Xanthophyll, Zeatin, Zeaxanthin, Zinc – Carotene- Alpha-Carotene, Beta-Carotene, Chlorophyll, Lutein, Neoxanthin, Violaxanthin, Xanthophyll, Zeaxanthin

Niacin has a relationship to normalizing cholesterol levels and increasing your metabolism as well as providing a little warmth on a cold winter's day. Winter's coming...Eat your Moringa.

Chronic Fatigue, Depression, Agoraphobia Testimonial

When I think back to one year ago, I was very low on many levels: no energy to do anything, 12 hours a day in bed and rest on the couch in the living room so I could see the sky outside. The only reason I moved to the couch was that a friend told me to get out of bed and find a place where you look at different surroundings. It was a major decision when I decided to take a shower every day, even though I was only able to sit on the stool in the shower, I would have horrible panic attack anxiety thinking that I was going to die based on how I felt. (I even messaged some people telling them this).

When the combination of anxiety and depression devastated me, I thought I would die, and I was convinced that no one would have anything to do with me. When I did have enough energy, I went to the store only at times when there were no people there because I developed anxiety to be in a crowded place or when people came too close. I had to have my phone on silent, and I could not listen to music, or watch TV with commercials. I read a great deal about this subject to tried and help myself because I loved music and being very active.

I learned about *Moringa oleifera* the summer when I was visiting with my daughter, and I began to take one packet per day on 19 July 2013. After 3 months there was a big change: I had lots of energy, my anxiety was gone, everything was no longer a *problem*. I was now very restless just sitting around and started back to work gradually over the winter being able to do 50% by January. Now it is good to live again!

In March 2014, I started taking two packages of Moringa per day, and it had a much better effect, so now I take 2 packs a day, and I expect to be 100% soon! In any case, I'm so good now that the problem is hardly noticeable anymore and I will now embark on a two-hour quick hike, and I look forward to listening to nature and enjoying life to the fullest.

Amino acid with promising anti-diabetic effects

PHARMACEUTICAL RESEARCH

New experiments conducted by researchers from the University of Copenhagen show that the amino acid arginine stimulates a hormone linked to the treatment of type 2 diabetes, and works just as well as several established drugs on the market. The research findings have just been published in the scientific journal *Endocrinology*.

More than 371 million people worldwide suffer from diabetes, of which 90% are affected by lifestyle-related diabetes mellitus type 2 (type 2 diabetes). In new experiments, researchers from the University of Copenhagen working in collaboration with a research group at the University of Cincinnati, USA, have demonstrated that the amino acid arginine improves glucose metabolism significantly in both lean (insulin-sensitive) and obese (insulin-resistant) mice.

"In fact, the amino acid is just as effective as several well-established drugs for type 2 diabetics," says Christoffer Clemmensen of the University of Copenhagen. He is currently conducting research at the Institute for Diabetes and Obesity at Helmholtz Zentrum München, the German Research Centre for Environmental Health in Munich.

To test the effect of the amino acid arginine, researchers subjected lean and obese animal models to a so-called glucose tolerance test, which measures the body's ability to remove glucose from the blood over time.

"We have demonstrated that both lean and fat laboratory mice benefit considerably from arginine supplements. In fact, we improved glucose metabolism by as much as 40% in both groups. We can also see that arginine increases the body's production of glucagon-like peptide-1 (GLP-1), an intestinal hormone which plays an important role in regulating appetite and glucose metabolism, and which is therefore used in numerous drugs for treating type 2 diabetes," says Christoffer Clemmensen, and continues:

"You cannot, of course, cure diabetes by eating unlimited quantities of arginine-rich almonds and hazelnuts. However, our findings indicate that diet-based interventions with arginine-containing foods can have a positive effect on how the body processes the food we eat."

The research findings were recently published in the American scientific journal *Endocrinology* under the heading *Oral l-arginine Stimulates GLP-1 Secretion to Improve Glucose Tolerance in Male Mice.*

Researchers have known for many years that the amino acid arginine is important for the body's ability to secrete insulin. However, the latest findings show that it is an indirect process. The process is actually controlled by arginine's ability to secrete the intestinal hormone GLP-1, which subsequently affects insulin secretion and "indicates a close biological connection between GLP-1 and arginine," says Christoffer Clemmensen, who conducted the biological experiments in the USA using a special animal model where the receptor for GLP-1 is genetically inactivated.

The new findings provide optimism for better and more targeted drugs for treating type 2 diabetes; the outlook is long-term but promising."

An interesting article but nevertheless this finding is not something new, and the arginine content in Moringa is substantial. More than 30% of *Moringa oleifera* is protein: amino acids and arginine numbers one of the twenty amino acids found in *Moringa oleifera*. The results of the work by Dr. Clemmensen is not something surprising to many of us.

Diabetes is an American epidemic. *Moringa oleifera* and the impact on diabetes would be an easy lecture topic to show the effectiveness of this phytonutrient dense plant. One of the most available areas for us to intervene and bring this potential crisis to a screeching halt is in serum glucose levels, and the work on arginine is only one mechanism.

Currently, in the US, there are approximately 26.1 million diabetics, and many of them have no idea that they are diabetic. Best estimates suggest that by 2050 there will be 130 million diabetics, indicative that this problem is out of control to such an extent that they have created a new category: pre-diabetic and instantly with these new diagnostic criteria there are 79 million prediabetics in America. This was the solution that was put forth. They have given up, but we know that a raw vegan diet will virtually eliminate Type 2 diabetes and one of the most powerful phytonutrient components to include in that diet is *Moringa oleifera*.

Diabetes & Cancer Testimonial

I am 52 years old, and I have used Moringa for almost one year now. Since 2006 I have been extremely ill, and I was diagnosed with latent autoimmune diabetes type 1 (LADA), an autoimmune variant. Two years later I was diagnosed with breast cancer, and there were serious complications that arose in the middle of chemotherapy when I got blood poisoning and an outbreak of Herpes (shingles). My medication seemed to create or reveal all kinds of other issues such as calcium poisoning and cataracts, and I was left with chronic fatigue syndrome exhaustion. My immune system was completely destroyed, and I was in so much pain that I was taking narcotic pain medication up to six times a day.

This downward spiral of health went on for several years while I was desperately trying to find something that could help me. In June 2013 I was introduced to Moringa, and finally, things started to happen quickly. My energy picked up, I slept better, the recurring outbreaks of shingles subsided, I have lost weight, my blood tests were better, and I use fewer insulin doses, but there is much more to my story.

January 2014 I underwent reconstruction surgery of the breast. My research indicated that I should increase my doses of Moringa, so I doubled them before and after the surgery. This time I did not get an infection in the wounds and outbreaks of shingles. My healing was amazing and overall health is now great! After one year, taking this Moringa formula is like getting the gift of life again. I take my Moringa every day with joy and have given up all other medications and supplements. My son at 20 is finally happy again, and we have hope for the future since my health is better. I am incredibly grateful for Moringa!

CHAPTER 7

Toxins Out Nutrients In 'Dirty Work'

So now that you have all this information about what is good for you and what is not, what will you do? I always talk about the steps that a person can take to shift from the chronological clock to the physiological clock. The first factor is always your diet but not in the way you might think...try not to hurt yourself with what you put into your body.

Most of you know who have been to my lectures know my thoughts on the food chain and the 10,000 chemicals that they can put into foods during preparation without telling you. The reason I mention diet is so that you try not to hurt yourself with what you eat. Is it any wonder that people consuming the correct varietal of *Moringa oleifera* start to detox very quickly.

The shelves are filled with chemicals masquerading as food, and the article below will ruin deep-fried foods for you. Read the article excerpts below or the whole article from the link. I was having a discussion today about toxins, and the process of detoxification and the bottom line is that no matter how unpleasant the detoxification process is, it is always better when the toxins are out of your body.

Acrylamide

To understand the nature of Pringles and other stackable chips, forget the notion that they come from actual potatoes in any recognizable way. The Pringles Company (in an effort to avoid taxes levied against "luxury foods" like chips in the UK) once even argued that the potato content of their chips was so low that they are technically not even potato chips. So if they're not made of potatoes, what are they exactly?

The process begins with a slurry of rice, wheat, corn, and potato flakes that are pressed into shape. This dough-like substance is then rolled out into an ultra-thin sheet cut into chip-cookies by a machine. "The chips move forward on a conveyor belt until they're pressed onto molds, which give them the curve that makes them fit into one another. Those molds move through boiling oil...Then they're blown dry, sprayed with powdered flavors, and at last, flipped onto a slower-moving conveyor belt in a way that allows them to stack. From then on, it's into the cans...and off towards the innocent mouths of the consumers."

Potato chips are one of the most toxic processed foods you can eat—whether they're made from actual potato shavings or not. One of the most hazardous ingredients in potato chips is not intentionally added, but rather is a byproduct of the processing.

Acrylamide, a cancer-causing, and potentially neurotoxic chemical is created when carbohydrate-rich foods are cooked at high temperatures, whether baked, fried, roasted or toasted. Some of the worst offenders include potato chips and French fries, but many foods cooked or processed at temperatures above 212°F (100°C) may contain acrylamide. As a general rule, the chemical is formed when food is heated enough to produce a fairly dry and brown/yellow surface. Hence, it can be found in: Potatoes: chips, French fries and other roasted or fried potato foods, grains: bread crust, toast, crisp bread, roasted breakfast cereals and various processed snacks, coffee; roasted coffee beans and ground coffee powder. Surprisingly, coffee substitutes based on chicory actually contains 2-3 times MORE acrylamide than real coffee. The federal limit for acrylamide in drinking water is 0.5 parts per billion or about 0.12 micrograms in an eight-ounce glass of water. However, a six-ounce serving of French fries can contain 60 micrograms of acrylamide or about FIVE HUNDRED times over the allowable limit.

Similarly, potato chips are notoriously high in this dangerous chemical. So high, in fact, that in 2005 the state of California actually sued potato chip makers for failing to warn California consumers about the health risks of acrylamide in their products. A settlement was reached in 2008 when Frito-Lay and several other potato chip makers agreed to reduce the acrylamide levels in their chips to 275 parts per billion (ppb) by 2011, which is low enough to avoid needing a cancer warning label.

The 2005 report "How Potato Chips Stack Up: Levels of Cancer-Causing Acrylamide in Popular Brands of Potato Chips," issued by the California-based Environmental Law Foundation (ELF), spelled out the dangers of this popular snack. Their analysis found that all potato chip products tested exceeded the legal limit of acrylamide by a minimum of 39 times, and as much as 910 times! Some of the worst offenders at that time included: Cape Cod Robust Russet: 910 times the legal limit of acrylamide, Kettle Chips (lightly salted): 505 times, Kettle Chips (Honey Dijon): 495 times."

http://www.antigmofoods.com/2013/07/cancer-in-can-what-you-need-to-know.html

Give The Body What It Needs Testimonial

My son was diagnosed with failure to thrive at 6 months old and borderline autism at 21 months old. We saw a Naturopath who put him on a number of homeopathic remedies. We fought yeast; we cut out sugar. He was fed organically from solid food introduction. After research, we determined that he had leaky gut. He wasn't absorbing any of his food. His diaper was full of chunks of the undigested food he ate, and the gastrointestinal specialist said that was normal. He was put on Miralax because supposedly he was holding his stools. He was also put on Prevacid for acid reflux.

We had upper and lower GI series x-rays done with no evidence of reflux found. However, the internist kept him on Prevacid. My boy cried non-stop. We tried different formulas, medicines. The biggest thing for him was and is sleep. He always went to sleep just fine but staying asleep was and is an issue. We went to another doctor and tried our best to give him 25 supplements three times a day at adult doses. It didn't change anything. I would call the doctor and say, "this supplement hasn't changed anything," and he would add more supplements never take any away. My boy hit his head constantly. He would spin in circles for 25-30 minutes without getting dizzy. He was still having meltdowns about 45% of his day. That's when I stumbled across *Moringa oleifera*. I began researching like a maniac.

My research led me to a proprietary *Moringa oleifera* formula, and I started him on it. I started noticing changes in him within a couple of weeks. Meltdowns were less, anger was less, and bowel movements were better. I was advised to give him D3 and another homeopathic supplement. I started those immediately, and I noticed a huge difference in his playing habits. He would play by himself more. He would actually watch an entire cartoon on television which he had never done before. His language went from 2-word sentences to 4-6 word sentences. Then I decided to take the homeopathic supplement away to see what happened. He was still playing; language was still exploding, watching his cartoons, happy, and no meltdowns. He's even gained a little weight.

Moringa oleifera has been an absolute answer to my prayers. My holistic physician said that the proprietary Moringa formula is the most bioavailable product he has seen in my 35 years of practice. I was so happy to finally have found the piece of the puzzle to my son's recovery. His anxiety is now in the past, and he is only 2.5 years old. It is amazing that all these changes have happened in three months taking Moringa.

There are choices to be made. Every health care professional in the world can only give you advice but it will always be your choice to be compliant. Do nothing and your life will go on pretty much as it is now. Take effective action in a proper sequence following a predictable empirically proven regimen and you will change everything forever.

CHAPTER 8

The Science of Exercise: Uncovering the Facts

> "Discovery consists of seeing what everybody has seen and thinking what nobody has thought."
>
> Albert Szent-Györgyi Nobel Prize Winner in Physiology or Medicine 1937, Discoverer of Vitamin C

As the science of exercise has continued to progress, many of the variable parameters of resistance training have been determined in order to maximize physical endurance and performance.[198][199] There are many physiological requirements to optimize physical performance from both the preparedness factor to the post-performance recovery factor that may be able to provide substrate and bioactive components to extend the overall benefits of physical activity.[200][201] "During post-exercise recovery, optimal nutritional intake is important to replenish endogenous substrate stores and to facilitate muscle-damage repair and reconditioning."[202] Energy, oxygen, electrolytes, minerals, hydration, antioxidants, anti-inflammatories, amino acids and even some carbohydrates will fill the requisite list.[203] [204] [205] Glucose and/or carbohydrates, amino acids and fatty acids can all be metabolized to produce energy in the form of ATP that can be utilized for protein synthesis.[206] In addition, amino acids are used directly for the synthesis of new proteins. A hydration source will be the vehicle to deliver the needed requirements.

The physiological importance of water cannot be overlooked. We may think of water superficially as the liquid that quenches our thirst, but this bi-polar fluid is responsible for hydrating cells, delivering nutrients, digestion, eliminating metabolic wastes, nutrient assimilation, respiration and maintaining the integrity of the total anatomy of the body. As a matter of fact, water is involved in every bodily function, and the proportion of body composition is staggering. Humans consist of approximately seventy to seventy-five percent (70%-75%) water. Human blood is approximately ninety-two percent (92%) water. The brain is roughly eighty-five percent (85%), and muscle tissue is seventy-five percent (75%) water respectively.[207] Any force that has the ability to affect water can affect the body and its functions, so it is imperative that optimize physiological function, water, or a viable substitute, is used as the carrier vehicle to deliver optimum nutrients.

Clearly to be prepared to perform in any task involves proper nutrition, proper training, and proper recovery and the above-mentioned components will not only enhance performance but maximize output on each and every occasion and for future events as well.[208] "Nutrient intake, before and after resistance exercise, alters the hormonal response and nutrient delivery and availability in skeletal muscle.... The balance of anabolic/catabolic hormones and the availability of nutrients (i.e., glucose and amino acids) will impact the regulation of carbohydrate, protein, and lipid balance. Over time, if this acute response to resistance exercise is of sufficient magnitude and duration, then protein accretion and muscle fiber hypertrophy will occur. The greater muscle mass will, in turn, increase expression of strength in subsequent workouts and affect the acute resistance exercise response."[209]

The above-stated conclusions by Dr. Jeff Volek, head of the Human Performance Laboratory at the University of Connecticut, give an excellent overview of the scientific literature concerning exercise physiology which is, in actuality the reason any and all athletes train. Furthermore, this body of knowledge sheds light on why *Moringa oleifera* is a totally effective nutrient source to optimize endurance, strength, and sport specific training. This African/Asian indigenous tree, commonly used for medicinal and nutritional purposes[210] is capable of delivering all the nutrition the body needs, and these enzymatically active amino acid sequences, antioxidants, omega fatty acids, and anti-inflammatories may simply not exist anywhere else in the food chain in this format, and that is just the tip of the nutritional iceberg when it comes to *Moringa oleifera*.[211,212,213]

Exercise has an unparalleled effect on muscle growth, and it can only happen when muscle protein synthesis is greater than muscle protein breakdown.[214,215] In the absence of amino acid intake in conjunction with the exercise regimen, net protein balance remains negative.[216,217,218] The timing, quantity, and quality of any nutritional intervention are the factors that will dictate the effectiveness of any routine.[219,220] Nutrient timing incorporates the specific regimen for eating of food and nutritional supplements. The intake scheduling and the ratio of the ingested nutrients are the factors that contribute to improved recovery, tissue repair, and muscle protein synthesis when compared to traditional strategies of nutrient intake.[221,222] Recovery is generally overlooked by the average individual who may not be training for an event or performance task, but the mindset has been changing over the last few decades as the exercise physiologists have explored all aspects of human conditioning.[223][224] The process of recovery actually begins at the onset of the physical task and includes protein intake. Protein and carbohydrate supplementation consumed before and after a resistance training session significantly contributes to the progress in exercise recovery.[225][226][227]

Amino acid ingestion directly following resistance exercise promotes skeletal muscle growth, and furthermore may be useful in neutralizing muscle wasting for conditions such as aging, cancer cachexia, physical inactivity, and rehabilitation following trauma or surgery.[228][229] Once the exercise/task has begun, the carbohydrate and fat fuels are the key sources of energy for the muscles respectively. Vigorous resistance training has been shown to have a positive effect on both muscle size and strength, increasing both the diameter and number of myofibrils with the result being increased size and strength.[230][231][232][233]

The next aspect of the physiological performance for consideration is to limit the potential damage that occurs as a result of the metabolic processes at hand. Muscles (myofibrils) are damaged or need immediate attention as the body tries to instantly repair, delay or prevent the onset of inflammation. Strenuous exercise causes muscles to be damaged, and subsequently, recovery becomes the process for muscular development and growth. "Resistance exercise substantially elevates protein turnover, and ingestion of essential amino acids before and after exercise stimulates transport of amino acids into skeletal muscle and protein synthesis."[234] Amino acid supplementation decreases myofibril damage and inflammation.[235][236]

A diverse spectrum of exercise brings about different changes to one's physiology and hence cross training for all athletic endeavors creates a more efficient, stronger body, able to use nutrition and oxygen better, offsetting the incidence of fatigue. All functions in the body are catalyzed by enzymes which are made of protein, vitamins, and minerals and are necessary for all aspects of metabolism. The increased rate of metabolism that occurs during exercise calls for increased production of enzymes.

Amino acids directly manage how efficiently the body functions and therefore the bioavailability of a complete essential amino acid source will ensure increased effectiveness for all biological reactions, especially muscular hypertrophy and strength increases from resistance exercise.[237][238][239] Endurance training or performance depletes the enzymes more quickly and the faster they can be replaced will optimize physiological function and decrease potential conversions to anaerobic mechanisms or inflammatory damage.

CHAPTER 9

Protein and Exercise

> "Nutrition is a valuable component that can help athletes both protect themselves and improve performance."
>
> *Bill Toomey, Olympic Gold Medalist*
> **1968 *Decathlon***

The main purpose of resistance training is that it results in an increase in overall strength and the size of muscle fibers. Muscle tissue is also made out of amino acids linked together, more commonly known as protein. There are nine essential amino acids that must be received from dietary sources since the human body cannot synthesize them (eight essential aa's for adults but histidine is also necessary for children). The essential amino acids are the following: isoleucine, leucine, lysine, methionine, phenylalanine, threonine, tryptophan and valine. Very few foods are known to contain all essential amino acids, hence, the importance of a phytonutrient like *Moringa oleifera*. As a matter of fact, *Moringa oleifera* is higher in amino acid content than legumes,[240] a source used by many vegetarians as their primary protein source.[241] How much protein synthesis occurs after exercise depends on the balance between the breakdown and the building of proteins. During the post-exercise phase, hormones such as testosterone and HGH are released to support and enhance this process of protein synthesis, this balance ultimately depends on available nutrients,[242] yet the relationship between nutrient input and hormonal response at this time remains unclear.[243]

To optimize athletic training and therefore output, the goal is to produce an ongoing environment in your body between workout sessions that diminish the breakdown of protein and increases protein synthesis.[244] All the essential amino acids must be present in the muscle in order for proteins to be made and limited availability of amino acids, enzymes and energy can decrease or eliminate protein synthesis.[245] The protein providing the amino acids, whether animal or vegetarian, does not matter from the actual muscle building perspective, as both sources were able to show a significant increase in increased muscle bulk and maximal dynamic strength.[246] Furthermore, there seems to be a greater benefit for strengthening and increasing the size of muscle if the amino acid supplement is available during the workout and can be consumed before,[247] and certainly as immediately as possible post workout.[248] [249] [250] Many of the amino acid formulae in the market offer products that are only to be consumed post-exercise, since their catabolic portions are quite high, utilizing these sources during a workout may reduce available blood for muscles. Unadulterated, enzymatically-active plants, however, can be consumed before and during exercise since they do not utilize significant physiological resources for digestion drawing blood borne resources away from muscles.

Vigorous workouts, stress, and fasting can initiate protein breakdown and cause the adrenal gland secretion of cortisol, a hormone released to reduce inflammation and consequently convert proteins to amino acids as an energy source. If cortisol levels remain elevated after exercise, protein breakdown continues and not only will muscle not be built, but it will be catabolized. Athletes who do not restore electrolytes and amino acids after exercise do not decrease cortisol levels. Foods with a high glycemic index will stimulate insulin release which will neutralize cortisol levels and minimize protein breakdown. The more complete a protein is in terms of the available essential amino acids, sequence and enzymatic activity will indicate the efficacy of performance and optimal physiological use. Many people are aware of the protein diets that have been promoted in recent times, and it is important to understand the digestive pathway for protein to understand how this works.

All nutrients ingested will follow either the anabolic or catabolic pathway. The designation associated with the biological value of a protein is the NNU, net nitrogen utilization. The NNU indicates the percentage of a protein that follows the anabolic (building) pathway versus catabolic pathway. Adulterated proteins tend to have lower anabolic indices whereas natural plant sources can be far more anabolic. *Moringa oleifera* should be considered to be the ultimate example of the former and more than adequately fulfills all needs in this category. This tree, which was named the NIH plant of the year in 2008, has such an abundant supply of amino acids that it is used to treat protein malnutrition and has been shown to improve overall nutritional status. [251] [252] [253] [254] [255] [256] [257] [258] [259]

After exercise, however, the limited availability of amino acids and energy is detrimental to both recovery and muscle growth and will limit protein synthesis. Borsheim et al. (2002) found that addition of a minimum of six grams of protein to the post-exercise carbohydrate supplement resulted in a net increase of protein uptake.[260] Moore et al. (2009), in a study published in the *American Journal of Clinical Nutrition*, identified 20 grams as the optimal amount of post-workout protein to maximize muscle growth.[261] Resistance exercise breaks down muscle requiring the replacement of amino acids to repair and increase muscle size (hypertrophy). The Moore study showed that more than 20 grams of protein after strenuous exercise does not build more muscle than the optimal amount. Volek (2004) who has explored the physiologic impact of dietary and exercise regimens and nutritional supplements, believes that to lift weights and not consume protein is virtually counterproductive.[262] Symons et al. (2009) found that the optimal amount of post-workout protein is no more than 30 grams and that protein added in excess of that does not increase strength or muscle bulk.[263] Conclusively protein (amino acids) is a necessary component to any exercise protocol, and one may safely assume that the dosage, somewhere around twenty (but less than thirty) grams dependent upon the quality of the protein.

Many foods, including nuts and beans, can provide a good dose of protein but it is crucial that the protein be complete, enzymatically alive, in the proper proportions and sequences. Animal protein is complete, but it takes a great deal of physiological energy to convert it to an available amino acid format, not to mention the diversion of metabolic enzymes for digestive functions. Many vegetarians create complete protein availability by combining legumes, nuts, and grains at one meal. *Moringa oleifera* is a complete protein containing all eight essential amino acids (including histidine) and the twenty amino acids found in the body.

Dr. Volek recommends splitting your dose of protein, consuming half thirty minutes before the workout and the other half thirty minutes post workout which makes *Moringa oleifera* an excellent source of protein to optimize this task. Less than one ounce of *Moringa* leaf powder provides forty-two percent (42%) of the recommended daily allowance of protein, more than all of the calcium requirements, sixty-one percent (61%) of the magnesium, forty-one percent (41%) of recommended potassium, almost triple the vitamin A (272%), seventy-one percent (71%) of the iron and twenty-two percent (22%) of the RDA for Vitamin C.[264] *Moringa oleifera* will soon become the protein source of choice for strength training and exercise of any kind based on the ratio and profile of available amino acids in conjunction with the bio-availability and presence of the physiological co-factors anti-inflammatories, antioxidants, carbohydrates, omega fatty acids, vitamins and minerals needed for optimal physiological benefit. Bird et al. (2006) have shown that combinations of nutrients such as amino acids and carbohydrates provide for greater muscle strengthening and growth.[265] The lack of available nutrients will limit the post-exercise protein synthesis progression. If the amino acids, vitamins, minerals and other nutritional components are not accessible when needed, the building stops, resulting in an inequitable muscular adaptation to benefits ratio. Protein requirements are directly related to their demographic parameters: sport, training intensity, and age of the participant.

CHAPTER 10

Optimizing For Peak Performance

"Now we know that there are good carbohydrates and bad carbohydrates. As science progresses and as public knowledge increases, the message becomes more complex."

James Dowd and Diane Stafford, Authors
'The Vitamin D Cure'

When athletes ingest carbohydrates during exercise, they are capable of oxidizing it at relatively high rates, sparing muscle glycogen depletion by up to 40% during the later stages of strenuous exercise and postponing fatigue.[266] [267] [268] The goal of exercise is to either train for performance, perform, or for conditioning. Carbohydrates are required to perform strenuous exercise, and their ingestion delays the onset of fatigue by up to forty-five minutes, making training more physiologically efficient. Carbohydrates during exercise maintain serum glucose levels to provide energy and should be ingested intermittently throughout the course of exercise.[269][270] "Currently scientific evidence suggests that carbohydrate supplementation prior to and during high-volume resistance training results in the maintenance of muscle glycogen concentration, which potentially could result in the maintenance or increase of performance during a training bout."[271] Optimal muscular glycogen stores can be best sustained by following a high-carbohydrate intake, and supplementation of free amino acids and protein alone or in combination with carbohydrate before resistance exercise can maximally stimulate protein synthesis.[272] Ingesting carbohydrates alone or in combination with amino acids during resistance exercise increases muscle glycogen, offsets muscle damage, and facilitates greater training adjustments.[273] On the basis of this information, it is advisable for athletes who are performing high-volume resistance training to ingest carbohydrate supplements before, during, and immediately after resistance training.[274][275] Carbohydrate ingestion following resistance exercise has been shown to enhance muscle glycogen re-synthesis decreasing recovery time and enabling an increase in the amount of training.[276][277][278] Supplying carbohydrate during exercise resulted in the postponement of muscular fatigue, allowing trained endurance athletes to oxidize the ingested carbohydrate at relatively high rates sparing muscle glycogen during the latter stages of prolonged strenuous exercise.[279][280]

Nazar et al. (1972) found that supplying carbohydrates during exercise delays the onset of muscular fatigue and increases endurance and strength in high-intensity exercise.[281] Studies have shown that *Moringa oleifera* leaves had the highest concentration when compared to widely used low glycemic index carbohydrates (110mg/ml) (10.1%).[282] Multiple authors conclude that *Moringa oleifera* contains ample amounts of bioavailable low caloric value carbohydrates, making it ideal as the carbohydrate source to utilize to maximize athletic training.[283][284][285][286] When considering both the carbohydrate content and protein content of *Moringa oleifera*, this plant has the ability to facilitate even greater adaptations to resistance training. [287][288]

Delayed Onset Muscle Soreness

Did you ever notice how quickly you breathe as you exercise? Exercise causes increased respiration as we urgently try to get more oxygen to our muscles. The body chooses to produce as much of its energy as possible aerobically with oxygen. When oxygen is limited, our bodies convert pyruvate into lactate, which permits glucose breakdown and this anaerobic energy production allows the working muscle cell to continue with intensity for up to several minutes. Lactate may build up to high levels and decrease the pH (acidity) of the muscle cells, disturbing physiology and severely limiting athletic ability.[289]

Contrary to urban legend, lactate or, as it is often called, lactic acid buildup is not responsible for the muscle soreness felt in the days following strenuous exercise. This recently dismissed theory conjectured that the accumulation of lactic acid as a consequence of vigorous exercise and the byproduct of muscle metabolism caused muscle soreness. Researchers have examined lactate levels immediately after exercise and discovered no significant correlation between the level of muscle soreness and lactic acid. This delayed-onset muscle soreness, (DOMS) occurs up to three days post-exercise and is characterized by varying levels of muscle tenderness in conjunction with decreased strength and diminished range of motion.[290] While the precise origin of DOMS remains unknown, current investigations lead to the source being muscle damage with concomitant catabolic metabolites in the tissue surrounding the muscle cells. These reactions to strenuous exercise result in an 'inflammatory-repair' response, with swelling and soreness at a maximum 48-72 hours post-trauma and usually resolving within a day or two depending on the nature of the damage.[291]

One of the best explanations for the cause of DOMS comes from Dr. Stephen M. Roth, a kinesiology professor, University of Maryland, "sore muscles are caused by microtrauma to the muscle fibers. When you overexert yourself physically, whether during work or play, you cause some localized irritation of the muscle fiber membranes, which can cause soreness. This pain can make it difficult to walk, reduce your strength, or make your life uncomfortable for a couple of days and is most likely caused by swelling in the muscle compartment from an influx of white blood cells, prostaglandins, histamines, nutrients and fluids that flow to the muscles to repair the 'damage' after a strenuous workout."[292] Some authors suggest that this delayed onset pain occurs when the inflammatory elements present in a muscle actually cause a physical pressure at nerve endings in the muscle.

Anti-inflammatories

It has been suggested that there are both pharmaceutical and nutritional solutions available to intervene in the DOMS problem. "Long-term supplementation with antioxidants or beta-hydroxy-beta-methyl butyrate appears to provide a prophylactic effect in reducing exercise-induced muscle damage (EIMD), as does the ingestion of protein before and following exercise."[293] Amino acid supplementation, when supplied post workout for up to 48 hours, eases DOMS and muscle damage.[294] Hasson et al. (1993) examined the effects of the anti-inflammatory (ibuprofen) on DOMS, and compared subjects given ibuprofen four hours before weight lifting (pre-lifting group) to subjects given ibuprofen twenty-four hours after lifting.[295] The pre-lifting ibuprofen group reported 40%

to 50% less soreness than the post-lifting ibuprofen group, demonstrating in this study that ibuprofen taken before exercise was more effective at reducing soreness than taking it after.[296] Cheung et al. (2003) investigated ibuprofen versus placebos taken every eight hours for 48 hours post-resistance exercise and found the ibuprofen group reported less soreness than the placebo group, proving that ibuprofen worked when taken after exercise.[297]

Although there is a diversity of reasons other than rigorous exercise, five and a half million people in the U.S. consume an analgesic, antipyretic, or nonsteroidal anti-inflammatory drug (NSAID) daily.[298] It should be noted that although anti-inflammatories decrease both the onset and duration of DOMS, ibuprofen and acetaminophen decreased the protein synthesis response that is normally seen after resistance exercise.[299] From these studies, it appears as if some people will respond to taking anti-inflammatories before working out, and others will respond when they take it afterward. When a plant containing broad-spectrum enzymatically-active natural anti-inflammatories is available, there will be the pain reduction without the decreased protein synthesis found with NSAIDs ibuprofen and acetaminophen. *Moringa oleifera* has thirty-six different anti-inflammatories and presents in a format that allows it to be easily consumed before, during and after resistance exercise.[300,301,302,303,304,305,306]

Antioxidants

Strenuous exercise is associated with a massive increase in whole-body oxygen uptake. Studies indicate that during vigorous exercise, reactive oxygen species (ROS) overpowers tissue antioxidant defense systems causing oxidative stress.[307] Exercise produces an increase in oxygen consumption reflecting the muscle's use of oxygen to provide energy in the form of adenosine triphosphate (ATP) and increases oxidative stress, adversely affecting exercise performance, and has been linked to increased fatigue, muscle damage and reduced immune function.[308][309][310][311] Increased oxygen utilization means an increase in the generation of free radicals, with the concerning result of muscle and tissue damage.[312][313][314][315] This muscular damage and fatigue, in all likelihood, will inhibit advancement in exercise training by impairing muscle recovery between exercise workouts, ultimately nullifying the reason for the exercise.

Anti-oxidants are substances that are generally ingested or produced by the body to provide electrons to bind with dangerous free radicals (ROS) and neutralize them. Free radical damage caused by electron-seeking, highly reactive, oxidative molecules with an unpaired electron has been identified as the source of many maladies through mechanisms such as inhibition of telomerase, changes to cellular permeability and DNA damage.[316]

Current evidence suggests that antioxidant supplementation reduces markers of oxidative stress associated with exercise.[317][318][319] McGinley (2009) found that mega-doses of antioxidants (Vit C, Vit E) may not be beneficial but the same could not be said for food source based antioxidants.[320] Sen (2001) suggests that a balanced diet, rich in foods with high antioxidant levels and supplements, is an athlete's best protection against the increased oxidative stress associated with strenuous exercise.[321] In essence, an athlete should increase their intake of antioxidant-rich foods (fruit and vegetables) to reflect their total energy/dietary intake. *Moringa oleifera* is one of the most antioxidant-rich foods on the planet, and it has been established that this phytonutrient dense tree contains forty-six different bioavailable anti-oxidants.[322][323][324][325][326][327][328]

Moringa oleifera contains antioxidants which may not only help with lean body mass gain but which can also promote other aspects of health. Antioxidant actions are believed to work against the onset and severity of many diseases, aging and health problems.[329][330] Intense or vigorous exercise depletes antioxidant capability and increases oxidant stress as determined in studies involving antioxidant capacity (plasma antioxidant status) and oxidative stress.[331][332][333] *Moringa oleifera* with the potent array of available antioxidants[334][335] has the distinct potential advantage of inhibiting two negative effects of training on antioxidant status: depletion of antioxidant capability and increased oxidative stress.[336][337]

The post-exercise ingestion of amino acids has been shown to stimulate vigorous increases in muscle protein synthesis, strength, and lean muscle development. When one adds a pre-exercise consumption of both amino acids and carbohydrates, it will result in peak levels of protein synthesis.[338][339] Furthermore, the addition of carbohydrates at all stages of the exercise regimen decreases fatigue and protects the levels of muscle glycogen.[340] If the amino acids, vitamins, minerals, and other building blocks are not present or available when they are required by the body, the anabolic process slows or stops completely.[341][342] *Moringa oleifera* contains close to one hundred nutrients, and according to the National Institute of Health, can cause the body to overcome more than three hundred diseases.[343] A proprietary *Moringa oleifera* formulation using the assorted parts of the tree contains the numerous nutrient complex factions of amino acids, antioxidants, anti-inflammatories, vitamins, minerals, omega 3-6-9 fatty acids, and low caloric value carbohydrates,[344] all in a bioavailable highly absorbable format that can provide all requisite nutrition. When following a workout supplementation regimen involving *Moringa oleifera*, this plant is able to provide all requisite nutrients for optimal physiological benefits that can be derived from training: maximal muscle growth, decreased muscle fatigue, increased muscle glycogen stores, decreased healing time, decreased post-workout muscle soreness (DOMS), and increased strength, guaranteeing optimal success for all endurance exercise endeavors.

As a researcher, I am continually asked, "What does this mean? What do I do with this theoretical information about a magical Moringa plant?" I will not shill for anyone because I always seek the best. I have empirically tested several Moringa products, and the results that I have found, point to three Moringa based products grown in a pristine manner and produced by a vertically integrated company that manufactures only pharmaceutical grade products (only need to be nutritional grade).

Effective protocols should be results-based, and I have been following my own protocol predicated by the science dictated by my research. The day before my sixty-second birthday, I was playing golf with a friend of mine who knew all about the drumstick tree. He was born and raised in India. When I golf, I walk. I carry my bag. This day, I shot a four-under-par, sixty-eight. I am hitting the ball farther off the tee since following my newly discovered protocol. My research indicates that if you can find the proper source for these products, you and the thousands of other athletes who have found it will achieve peak performance.

PART III

Moringa Applied

CHAPTER 11

So Now What?

"What do I do with this theoretical information about a magical Moringa plant?"

Narrator: What if you are like Gary (who has been ailing of some chronic disease—who may or may not have been diagnosed with stage 4 cancer) here and you just slept through the health lecture—you missed Dr. Fisher's brilliant discussion of the science of Moringa?

Gary: Well actually I wasn't sleeping—I was watching the Reds-Cubs game on my phone.

Narrator: So wait, let me get this straight—you are DYING of "Dis-Ease," and you were too busy watching a baseball game to listen to a guy tell you about a plant that could save your life?

Gary: Well, when you put it that way, it kinda sounds bad...but if the Reds win 50 of their last 55 games, they could still maybe get the wild card.

Narrator: Dude, you're dying! And you care more about watching people on TV playing a meaningless game than you do about living your own life!

Gary: Ok, you might be right. Can you give me the "Cliff Notes" version?

Narrator: Actually, I might have a better idea. Maybe we try the Mary Poppins approach?

Gary: You mean a spoonful of sugar to make the medicine go down?

Narrator: No, but a spoonful of raw organic cane sugar might help the Moringa go down. Someone should write that song. Actually, I was thinking more along the lines of "Find the fun, and the job's a game." Maybe we could come up with something like, "Who wants to be a health-o-naire?"

Gary: Can't we just stick to "Who wants to be a millionaire?"

Narrator: Man, who cares if I give you a million bucks if you are dying of...

Gary: Well, I don't know this Fisher guy, how do I know he's telling the truth?

Narrator: Well, didn't you hear him cite all the research, those PubMed articles, etc.? Oh wait, that's right, you were too busy listening to that life-changing ballgame.

Gary: Yeah but I also saw a great advertisement for a new drug that might help my condition.

Narrator: Did you listen to the side effects?

Gary: Side effects? All I saw were the happy, smiling energetic people!

Narrator: And of course you trust those actors. Maybe that's your problem—the food you eat, the advice you take.

In whom do you trust?
Doc Fisher has done a phenomenal job presenting the science of Moringa…why it matters. What I like is that he's done the research, gone through all the data, so I don't have to. All I have to do is listen to his breakdown of the information and ask the right questions. Does this comport with my worldview? Does this make sense? Well, for me, it did. I believe that as the Bible says: 1) "God created the heaven and the earth;" 2) God made me "fearfully and wonderfully"; and 3) God made plants including this most nutrient-dense plant called Moringa to nourish me. So it was a simple logical deduction, and now I have seen the tremendous results for myself and my family. In addition to the numberless health benefits of taking the most nutrient-dense plant ever discovered, the financial benefits are enormous. Moringa is without a doubt, the best "nutritional bang for the buck" and has saved me countless dollars.

However, that's irrelevant to you. It doesn't matter what I think or what I tell you to do if you aren't convinced for yourself, and it's much more than simply saying you are convinced. A lot of people say they believe things and yet never put them into practice. I've known far too many people who say they believe Moringa works and yet they don't take it. Some even order it and let it sit on their shelf. Some even mix it up and put it in the fridge but stunningly, never drink it. Some drink it for a little bit and then, it just stops being convenient.

Back to the highway analogy Doc used—he tells you "don't go play in the traffic." Most people would trust that opinion to be pretty good advice regardless of who gives it. It just seems like common sense to not play in the middle of a busy highway. You really don't even need a statistic to tell you that 95 out of every 100 people that play in traffic for more than 15 consecutive minutes end up getting hit (FACT CHECK– this is not an actual proven statistic). The stat simply confirms for you what "logic dictates." I love that phrase "logic dictates" which Howie uses often, as do I. See, I love the game of chess which I believe is the greatest game of logic. You must ask logical questions before making a move which may lead to a winning combination as well as potential disaster.

If I play in traffic, am I more likely than not to be hit by a car? Yes. Are there any advantages to playing on that busy highway? Do they outweigh the potential risks? If they do, go for it! But I'm guessing we all agree or at least the vast majority that no good can come from risking playing in heavy traffic on Highway 401 or any highway for that matter.

So without further ado, let's play a game in which we will have questions and answers which will hopefully allow us to arrive at a most logical and satisfactory conclusion.

CHAPTER 12

"THIS AIN'T JEOPARDY"
But your life may be in it!

Announcer: Good evening folks and welcome to "This Ain't Jeopardy" but as we like to say here on the show; "your life may very well indeed be in jeopardy." So think of this as a chess game. As someone once observed, "life is a kind of chess." It's made of many moves, and we must ask the important questions with each move. "What is this move doing? What is this move no longer doing? Is this move making my position better or worse?" Of course, remembering our "end game," we must ask: "Is this move getting me closer to my objective or is it causing me to drift aimlessly and will it lead to disaster if not corrected?"

Now here are the hosts of "This Ain't Jeopardy," Dr. Howard Fisher and Steve Wilson also known as "the doctor and the dummy."

Steve: Kind of insulting you might think but we're all dummies about something, right? After all, there is that whole book series, but I've yet to see "Moringa for Dummies" so this is as close as we may get. "Moringa for Morons" maybe? How bout we just do what my good friend Howie always reminds me when I'm trying to tell somebody about Moringa. "Keep it simple Steve!" Contestants on "This Ain't Jeopardy" will do well to remember that and pay attention to any other interjections by Dr. Fisher...like this one below....

Howie: My friend Russ Bianchi loves to explain a diversity of seemingly inexplicable phenomena with the following quote referencing Ockham's Razor, "Invariably the simplest answer tends to be the correct one," as suggests. The simple answer, in this case, is the industrialized, processed, chemically refined, and genetically modified food and beverage chain, along with a tsunami of harmful drugs, is killing us. We are overfed, undernourished, and over- drugged."

Announcer: You can't put it any more succinctly than that. Now let's meet our contestants whose names have been changed to protect their identities. To stick with the KISS acronym, we've named our contestants—Scott, Seymour and Sophia. Scott is a sports-obsessed, TV-loving, fast-food junkie who makes little or no time for his health. Scott refuses to think for himself and can't fathom that the government or the "talking heads" might lie to him. Seymour is a health activist and amateur conspiracy theorist and very opinionated about both. Sophia is a serious and mild-mannered young woman with a keen interest in learning what she can do to be more healthy.

Host: Thank you for joining us today on "This Ain't Jeopardy." Remember contestants, the simplest answer is usually the correct one so just remember the name of the category and think of the appropriate question.

Scott: (Turning to Seymour) What did he say?

Seymour: It doesn't matter. You've already lost. Just listen to what I say, and you might learn something.

Sophia thinks to herself, *"These guys are clueless. All I have to do to win is remember the three R's— 'Reading, Reasoning and Responsibility.' Read the answer carefully. Reason effectively— does this make sense? Then take responsibility and answer in the form of a question."*

Host: Let's take a look at the categories for Round 1. They are as follows: Killing Us; Conspiring to Kill Us; That's SAD; GMO's; That's a Great Question; and SAY WHAT?!

Let's begin, and we will go through the categories in logical order.

(Things that are) KILLING US:

100- Inflammation is the common denominator of many chronic age-related diseases such as arthritis, gout, Alzheimer's, and diabetes.

Seymour: And yet they don't want to do anything about it. Just prescribe more drugs that cause more side effects and harm to people instead of looking at natural alternatives.

Host: Seymour, please put your answer in the form of a question.

Scott: What do you mean "they?" Who is "they?"

Host: That was in the form of a question but not the answer we're looking for.

Howie: The literature has been filled with the relationship between inflammation and chronic disease and suggests that as much as 80% of all chronic disease is directly due to inflammation.

Sophia: What are "things that are killing us?"

Host: Correct Sophia! We would also accept simply, "what is killing us?"

200- Food no longer works! If it did, we would be able to use it to keep our bodies functioning properly...

Seymour: That's abominable! Food used to work! Why does it not anymore?! What are they doing to the food supply?!

Scott: There you go with "they" again—who is they? What are you—some kind of conspiracy nut?

Host: Sorry, neither of you provided the answer we were looking for.

Sophia: What is "killing us?"

Host: Yes, Sophia. Correct for 200 Moringa Reward points!

300- Studies that compared the mineral content of soils today (1992) with soils 100 years ago (1892) found that agricultural soils in the United States have been depleted of eighty-five percent (85%) of their minerals.

Seymour: Did you hear that—85%?!

Host: Sorry, that was in the form of a question but not the one we were looking for.

Scott: But the food sure does taste better! (Scott takes a bite of a donut.)

Sophia: What is "killing us?"

Host: Correct for 300 reward points!

Howie: Do you think it is getting better or worse…twenty-two years later?

400- Everything you ingest, inhale or absorb must be sorted out by your immune system or liver, and consequently, your liver is overworked. With only four venues of detoxification (skin, lungs, urinary or fecal) often times your body is unable to dispose of the vast amount of toxins in our environment.

Seymour: That's right Scott. Those donuts you're ingesting are killing you! You're overworking your liver! What is wrong with you?!

Howie: Seymour, remember share don't push.

Scott: But the donuts; they taste so good. How can they be bad for me?

Sophia: What is "killing us?"

Host: Yes, that is absolutely correct for 400 more Moringa reward points!

500- There are billions of pounds of more than 100,000 different toxic chemicals released into the environment annually. Forty-two billion pounds of toxic chemicals either manufactured or imported into the US daily.

Seymour: These people are despicable! They want us all dead! There's your simple answer!

Host: Unfortunately, Seymour, it's the wrong answer, and it wasn't in the form of a question.

Scott: Why do you keep saying, "they"? Who is "they"? Who do you think is killing us?

Host: Scott, that was three questions, but unfortunately none of them were correct.

Sophia: What is "killing us?"

Howie: Would you be surprised to know that almost 10 years ago they sampled umbilical cord blood in newborns and found an average of 287 chemicals in each newborn? Of the 287 chemicals we detected in umbilical cord blood, we know that 180 cause cancer in humans or animals, 217 are toxic to the brain and nervous system, and 208 cause birth defects or abnormal development in animal tests. The dangers of pre- or post-natal exposure to this complex mixture of carcinogens, developmental toxins and neurotoxins have never been studied. **Face it! If you're not detoxing, you're toxic.**

Host: Thank you for elaborating Dr. Fisher. Outstanding job Sophia! You swept that category and earned 1500 Moringa reward points. Seymour and Scott, remember that often the simple answer is the correct one.

Conspiring To Kill Us:
100- *"I have arrived at a conclusion so alarming and urgent that it can only be stated bluntly. Based on what I am seeing via atomic spectroscopy analysis of all the dietary substances people are consuming on a daily basis, I must now announce that the battle for humanity is nearly lost. The food supply*

appears to be intentionally designed to end human life rather than nourish it." Mike Adams...Natural News

Seymour: They aren't going to stop until they murder us all! We must hold these people accountable!

Scott: Who is "they?" Who are "these people?"

Host: Please be more specific.

Scott: Who is "conspiring to kill us?"

Host: That's correct! (Surprised tone) You just earned 100 Moringa reward points!

Howie: The food chain has been broken, and whether it has been done deliberately or not, the fact remains that it is.

Seymour: Well, we know it is deliberate! How else could you possibly explain it!

Howie: Remember, let them come to their own conclusions.

200-"With *Salt Sugar Fat: How the Food Giants Hooked Us*, Pulitzer Prize-winning investigative journalist Michael Moss has laid out the foundation and blueprints of the inevitable future raft of class action lawsuits targeting the food industry for knowingly and scientifically designing products that encourage their over-consumption despite their known and well-understood risks."

Seymour: See that's what I've been saying! it's these greedy, unscrupulous corporations that are putting profits before people and systematically undermining our food supply. They don't care how many people they hurt or kill as long as they can make money doing it!

Scott: But they make it taste so GOOD! How can it be bad for us?

Host: Oh sorry, Scott. That's incorrect.

Seymour: See, he still doesn't get it.

Host: You can't buzz in twice, Seymour. And again, that wasn't a question.

Sophia: Who is "conspiring to kill us?"

Host: Correct again, Sophia. You have earned another...

Howie: I think the readers get the point. Every time someone asks the right question, they get a reward. If they follow those questions to their logical conclusion, they get an even bigger reward.

Host: Well said. So you're telling me I don't have to keep saying how many Moringa reward points they have earned?

Howie: I think they will be able to figure out that there are logical consequences for their actions and hopefully adapt their thinking and behavior accordingly.

300- The truth of the matter is that natural alternatives do not even receive nearly as much funding as pharmaceutical drugs and medical interventions because there's simply no room for profit.

Seymour: See, there you have it! It's all about the money—follow the money, and you'll get your answer on who is behind the plan to exterminate us! They don't want us to be healthy. Because there's no profit in having people healthy!

Scott: But there is profit in making great donuts! (He takes another bite).

Host: Oh sorry, Scott that will cost you 300 Moringa points but if you keep eating those donuts, it will cost you much more—maybe even your life.

Howie: Let him figure that out for himself, and I told you to stop with the points. There is much more at stake here. Don't confuse people. Don't be short-sighted. Achieving health is its own reward. If you get reward points, that's "Moringa gravy." (Note to reader: Howie didn't use the phrase "Moringa gravy" which doesn't actually exist—I threw that in).

Scott: Can you put Moringa gravy on biscuits? I might could go for that.

Sophia: Who is "conspiring to kill us?"

400- The real mystery is how this five-thousand-year-old panacea plant went missing and disappeared from the nutritional horizon.

Seymour: Who are the same guys that made the "flat earth" disappear?

Host: Oh, sorry. Wrong conspiracy.

Howie: Do you not think that it is extremely interesting that most people on the planet have never heard of *Moringa oleifera*. Do you think that there may be other agendas in place? How is it possible that the most phytonutrient dense plant that had been in use for 5000 years vanished? Perhaps it is time to look at preventative measures.

Scott: What is he talking about?

Sophia: Who is "conspiring to kill us?"

500- However, it really grates me to see efficacious formulations or products dumb-downed, or intentionally blocked from use, by greedy, stupid, and unscrupulous economic marketers, once delivered for production or distribution.

Seymour: Yeah, even the people out there pretending to be our friends. Even the people out there claiming to make "health" products. When I think of all the good money that I've wasted on vitamins and supplements that don't even work! Or worse—those that are actually harming me and my family!

Howie: Over the counter vitamins (poo poo pellets) usually end up untouched in the toilet due to their glycol coatings so they don't work and vitamins need minerals to function.

Scott: So see, it's not just the people making good donuts; it's your health-nut friends as well conspiring against us. There's nothing we can do so we might as well watch TV.

Sophia: Who is "conspiring to kill us?"

THAT'S SAD (Standard American Diet or...):
100- Convenience and the average western diet are leading us down a path that leads right over a cliff: metabolic syndrome

(obesity, inflammation, diabetes, and coronary heart disease) and early death.

Scott: Wait—that question is not an attack on America is it? We invented convenience and the world owes us! Fast food, the microwave, and the DVR feature—how did we ever survive without these?

Seymour: Scott, are you insane?! He said convenience is leading us down the path over a cliff! Are you too stupid to stop a lifestyle that is going to kill you?!

Howie: Seymour, remember share don't push.

Sophia: What is "that's SAD?"

200- Poor nutrition has been linked to the major chronic diseases, immune system dysfunction and premature aging that are affecting the global population leading to a decreased quality of life.

Scott: Yeah but my grandma is 95 years old, and she doesn't eat much better than I do.

Seymour: Again can you not read? It's quality-of-life, not quantity—there's a big difference! Do you just want to sit in the chair and wait to die? Well, I guess you could still watch your ball games and eat your fast food...

Host: Seymour, please remember to answer in the form of a question and direct your comments towards the host, not to the other contestants.

Sophia: What is "that's SAD?"

300- The common North American diet is pro-inflammatory by a significant ratio of Omega Fatty Acids alone. Omega 6 is inflammatory and should have a ratio of 2:1 with Omega 3 which is anti-inflammatory. The typical western diet has a ratio of approximately 20:1 which predisposes those of us to chronic disease and increased aging.

Seymour: Wow, that is so sad.

Host: Oh, closer but still not in the form of a question.

Sophia: What is "that's SAD?"

400- We have a good idea what are the factors in major diseases and the solutions to these are absent from our food chain…all while decreasing the soils' quality with abusive farming practices—most veggies and fruits grown today now contain way fewer nutrients than 50 years ago."

Scott: OK you said that already, didn't you? We get it—the food chain is broken, but it still tastes AMAZING!

Seymour: (Frowning, shaking his head)

Host: Um, I will need to ask the judges about that. Sorry, our judges are unable to accept facial expressions as a correct response.

Sophia: What is "that's SAD?"

500- Somewhere around January-February, we may not see much of the sun in northern climates, and that is when depression strikes in the form of "this…." It is believed that people are adversely affected by the decreasing amounts of sunlight and the colder temperatures as the fall and winter progress. This is probably a relationship between Vitamin D, which aids in absorption of all nutrients and the physiological implications leading to the symptoms: depression, fatigue, irritability, difficulty concentrating, decreased sex drive, poor sleep, decreased activity level, increased pain, and carbohydrate craving.

Scott: Yeah I hate cold weather, but at least it's a good excuse to stay inside, watch TV and order pizza and wings!

Seymour: (Rolling his eyes) What is "Stupid Affective Disorder?"

Host: Sorry, no.

Sophia: What is "SAD?"

Host: That's right and in this case meaning "Seasonal Affective Disorder."

GMOs:
100- It's not rocket science to understand that when you eat a steady diet of these horrible chemicals, you will suffer disastrous health ramifications.

Scott: What are polyphenols?

Host: Oh sorry, no.

Seymour: Didn't you listen to anything Dr. Fisher said? Polyphenols are good for you!

Sophia: What are "GMOs?"

200- These foods are not good for our health. There is so much proof in this department; it is insulting that Monsanto would tell us otherwise. The French have proven GMO causes cancer.

Scott: Well, you can't trust the French. If it ain't made in America, I don't buy it, and I don't need no Europeans snobs telling me how and what to eat.

Seymour: I hate "Monsatan!"

Sophia: What are "GMOs?"

300- Russia will not import these products, the country's Prime Minister Dmitry Medvedev said, adding that the nation has enough space and resources to produce organic food.

Scott: Can't trust the Russians either.

Seymour: What is the end game?

Host: We will give you partial credit for that answer.

Sophia: What are "GMOs?"

400- "If the Americans like to eat these products, let them eat it then. We don't need to do that…

Scott: Well we ought to drop a nuke on them. Those condescending Commies!

Seymour: So, who really won the cold war? Howie said it best—"looks like they beat us to the freedom of information act." It should sicken us that in the "land of the free and home of the brave," we have lost a much more important war to the

Russians—the health war! The war over GMO foods and the right to have our food labeled! We are worried about outside threats while the "powers that be" in our own country are deceiving us and leading us like lambs to the slaughter. Maybe we should spend at least equal time dealing with the enemies within our borders?

Host: Valid points but please answer in the form of a question and let others draw their own conclusions.

Sophia: What are "GMOs?"

500- So the question to ask is 'what are the other governments waiting for' (to ban these)?

Seymour: Well, that's a great question!

Scott: We shouldn't do anything the Russians would do!

Sophia: What are "GMOs?"

THAT'S A GREAT QUESTION:
100- What are they doing to your produce?

Seymour: Again, another great question!

Scott: Who is "they?" The French?!

Sophia: What is "that's a great question?"

200- Have they known that plants offer the solution to health?

Seymour: Of course THEY do! But they can't patent a plant! Follow the money!

Sophia: What is "that's a great question?"

300- Monsanto Has Been Removed And Banned By: Austria, Bulgaria, Germany, Greece, Hungary, Ireland, Japan, Luxembourg, Madeira, New Zealand, Peru, South Australia, Russia, France, and Switzerland! Is your country on this list? Why Not?

Scott: No, cause we're smarter than all those countries. We must have some good reason for it, but we're not gonna share it with them.

Sophia: What is "that's a great question?"

400- To understand the nature of Pringles and other stackable chips, forget the notion that they come from actual potatoes in any recognizable way. The Pringles Company (in an effort to avoid taxes levied against "luxury foods" like chips in the UK) once even argued that the potato content of their chips was so low that they are technically not even potato chips. So if they're not made of potatoes, what are they exactly?

Scott: I don't know, and I don't care. They taste great!

Seymour: What is what you don't know may be killing you?

Sophia: What is "that's a great question?"

500- Is society taking a serious approach to disable disease or is the agenda to disable society? Diabetes is not going away which when we examine the Moringa literature seems ridiculous. How is it that this serum glucose insulin disorder, especially diabetes 2, has become so totally out of control?

Seymour: Follow the money!

Scott: Do donuts cause diabetes?

Sophia: What is "that's a great question?"

Howie: There are now 79 million prediabetics in America. This was the solution that was put forth. With no sign of being able to change this downward spiral to diabetes, they merely created a new category. They have given up. **If the powers that be really wanted to get rid of the problem.... Well, you can just come to your own conclusion.**

SAY WHAT?!:
100- Monsanto claims that GMOs are safe.

Seymour: Those lying...did I mention that I hate Monsatan?!

Sophia: What is "SAY WHAT?!"

200- The liver is the workhorse of our bodies and it is bad enough that they have to deal with the four billion pounds (that's right 4,000,000,0000) of toxic chemicals dumped into the North American environment annually and the ten thousand of chemical additives put into our food supply that they do not have to tell you about.

Scott: Would they do that? By North American, do you mean the Canadians? America wouldn't do that.

Seymour: Of course they would. You'd know that if you stopped watching so much TV! Stop being brainwashed and start thinking for yourself!

Sophia: What is "SAY WHAT?!"

300- Currently, it is illegal for any food, herb, tincture or superfood product to say that it cures anything, yet medications advertised on TV since 1997 can say they treat all kinds of diseases and disorders, even though the side effects are horrendous, some of the time including internal bleeding and suicide.

Scott: But the people in the drug commercials are always smiling. Why would they smile if there are side effects to the medication or if it was bad for us?

Seymour: I give up.

Sophia: What is "SAY WHAT?!"

400- Best estimates suggest that by 2050 there will be 130 million diabetics which suggests that this problem is out of control to such an extent that they have created a new category: pre-diabetic. There are now nearly eighty million prediabetics in America. This was the solution that was put forth. With no sign of being able to change this downward spiral to diabetes, they merely created a new category. Very recently the estimates have been upgraded in an extremely negative way: by 2020 50% of the US population will be diabetic or prediabetic. They have given up.

Scott: There you go with the "they" again. Who is "they?"

Seymour: Just blame it on the Russians, Scott. Like "they" told you on TV.

Sophia: What is "SAY WHAT?!"

500- Moringa is too expensive…

Scott: What is Moringa?

Seymour: Not what, who? He's that shortstop for the Reds.

Scott: What? We got a new shortstop. I didn't hear that.

Seymour: We? Do you play for the Reds? No, you don't, but you invest more of your time in them than you do taking care of your own health.

Sophia: What is "SAY WHAT?!"

Howie: So you say you cannot afford to take Moringa and I say the evidence is overwhelming that you cannot afford to not take it. Mike Adams, The Health Ranger, expressed it perfectly when he said, "You can't put a price tag on being healthy.… It's priceless."

Host: That's absolutely correct! Now it's time for the second round of "This Ain't Jeopardy" which focuses on the solution to some of the problems we've been discussing. Of course, when we talk solutions, we must start from the ultimate beginning, so our categories begin with God. Then we have Dr. Howard Fisher; You; Your Body; The Prevention is the Cure; and Moringa Oleifera.

THE SOLUTION

GOD:

100- *According to the Westminster Shorter Catechism, "(He) is a spirit, infinite, eternal, and unchangeable, in his being, wisdom, power, holiness, justice, goodness and truth.* [345]

Scott: What is mother nature?

Seymour: Good grief.

Host: No, sorry.

Sophia: What is "God?"

200- Genesis 1:1 says, "In the beginning (He) created the heaven and the earth."

Scott: Does that include TV?

Seymour: Seriously?

Sophia: What is "God?"

300- Genesis 1:27 says "So (He) created man in his *own* image…male and female created he them.

Scott: Wait, there are only two genders?

Seymour: Well, if you turned off the TV and opened a Bible, you might know that.

Howie: Share, don't push.

Sophia: What is "God?"

400- In Genesis 1:29 (He) said the following: "Behold, I have given you every herb bearing seed, which *is* upon the face of all the earth, and every tree, in which *is* the fruit of a tree yielding seed; to you, it shall be for meat."

Seymour: That's right, he's a good and wise Creator who gives good gifts—"every good and perfect gift" in fact. If you would just take a little bit of your most precious asset, your time and study God's Word, you might arrive at different conclusions than what you hear on television.

Host: Thank you, Seymour, for the much more compassionate response but unfortunately...

Seymour: I know, I know...not in the form of a question. I hate that part of this game.

Sophia: What is "God?"

500- Exodus 15:25 says that He "shewed (Moses) a tree, *which* when he had cast into the waters, the waters were made sweet: there he made for them a statute and an ordinance, and there he proved them..."

Scott: But the tree was discovered in America, right? Moses was American.

Seymour: No, it wasn't, and he wasn't. While we can't say for sure exactly what tree it was, we do know who made the tree and that He gave it as a good gift to his creation to make those waters sweet. It could have, in fact, even been a "miracle tree."

Sophia: What is "God?"

Dr. Howard Fisher:
100- I live in Toronto, Canada and we have one of the largest busiest highways in the world, Highway 401, which has more than sixteen lanes at some points, and there is always traffic.

This services the metropolitan population of approximately seven million people. My responsibility to the patient is to give advice, and if I were to warn them not to play in the middle of this highway because they might get hurt, I have carried out my responsibility. If they do and they get hurt, I have done all that I can do. If they were to run into a problem and I also gave advice which resolved the problem it is very much the same thing.

Sophia: Who is "Dr. Fisher?"

Host: Yes, we also would have accepted Doc Fisher.

200- I have been doing anti-aging research for over 30 years and have advocated the relationship between nutrition and intervention in the disease/aging complex for nearing three decades.

Sophia: Who is "Dr. Fisher?"

300- For decades now I would say to my patients, "Try not to hurt yourself with what you eat, but try to get your nutrition somewhere."

Howie: I have taken the liberty of modifying Hippocrates' adage, "Give the body what it needs, and the body will repair itself to the best of its ability. If you give the body Moringa, those abilities increase."

Sophia: Who is "Dr. Fisher?"

400- I have been on this preventive approach for thirty years, and now they realize how important diet and environment are. I think perhaps the introduction of a phytonutrient dense plant would be the perfect intervention.

Sophia: Who is "Dr. Fisher?"

500- Some people watch TV, but for me, TV is background noise while I read journal papers. I thought I might just appeal to the interesting side of being a researcher, so you know why I answer questions the way I do. Someone once asked me how many papers I have read about *Moringa oleifera*...it is a number with at least three zeroes.

Sophia: Who is "Dr. Fisher?"

YOU:
100- It is apparent that if there was a 'State of the Food Chain Address,' that ___ would want to make changes to improve your health with this knowledge.

Scott: Well, I would listen if there wasn't a game on.

Seymour: Scott, you just keep forsaking your own mercy. I actually am starting to pity you. When I think about it, I used to be a lot like you too, and I wouldn't listen either. In fact, I still don't listen like I should and let my pride get in the way of helping people like you...people like me.

Sophia: Who is "you?"

Host: Correct! We will also accept, "who are you?"

200- More than thirty years of treating patients and listening to the plethora of reasons for lack of compliance has made me realize that I can only offer guidance and that any form of implementation in a free society rests with ___.

Scott: We the people!

Seymour: Yes, we are free to make choices, but too often they are misinformed and contrary to sound reason. "So it's not about the fight. It's not about being right." It's about being humble and sharing what you know to be true. Which begs the question, how do we know what is true? What is our objective standard for truth?

Host: That's a good question but not the one we were looking for here.

Sophia: Who is "you?"

Seymour: But how do "you" or "I" make the right choices? We have to go back to "first principles." We have to have some clear rationale guiding us to make good decisions when we are being lied to, manipulated and being led astray or into paralyzing fear by "they."

Scott: WHO ARE THEY?!

Seymour: Do you really want to know?

Scott: I want the truth!

Seymour: Can you handle the truth?

Host: Save it for after the show, guys or for another book. Back to the board.

300- It definitely seems to me that if you are aware of a non-GMO nutrient source and you do not make it a part of the protocol, that some of the blame lies with ____!

Scott: The...Russians?

Seymour: Well, at least you hesitated.

Scott: Yeah, well, I'm starting to question whether maybe the Russians infiltrated our government and...

Host: Sophia...

Sophia: Who is "you?"

400- With no sign of being able to change this downward spiral to diabetes, they merely created a new category. They have given up. ____ have just been handed the ball.

Scott: Is it a baseball or basketball?

Seymour: That's not the point. The point is that...

Host: Sophia...

Sophia: Who is "you?"

Seymour: You can't blame your poor choices on the Russians or expect that your government, the media or your doctor is going to save you. In fact, they might just be lying to you as hard as that is for you to accept.

500- It has already been demonstrated that no agency will safeguard your health better than____.

Scott: Wait, I think I might know this one…is it me?

Seymour: Yes, it's you!

Host: Well, you're both half-right. Sophia…

Sophia: Who are "you?"

Host: Yes, that's the point of this category. The point of this show, or the point of this book, we present information, you must ask the right questions and come to your own conclusions.

Howie: This book will be exactly that, please feel free to read the articles, many of which are taken directly from the source and footnoted so you can easily find them. There are many opinions expressed here, both my own and those of hundreds of other researchers and authors so feel free to accept what you will and disregard the rest. You may find many facts repeated…let the impact sink in because these statistics are important as they reflect how things have escaped our control.

YOUR BODY:
100- Psalm 139:14 says that "it" is "fearfully and wonderfully made."

Seymour: What is "your body?"

200- Hippocrates adage about giving "it" what it needs and letting it correct itself…

Scott: What is "your body?"

Host: Wow! Well guys, better late than never! Welcome to the game!

300- The food chain is broken, and it is time to give "it" the nutrition "it" needs.

Scott: What is "your body?"

Host: YES!

Scott: And you're sure there's no nutrition in donuts?

Seymour: The better question might be: "Did God make donuts or GMO foods to fuel your fearfully and wonderfully made body?

Scott: That's a good question though a hard one.

Sophia: All the best questions are hard. But the answers are usually simple!

Howie: Your body will extract 90-95% of the nutrition in an enzymatically alive plant because that is what your body was designed to do...extract nutrition, when available, from a food source. The more natural the food source, the more nutrient dense the food source, the easier it is.

400- Our second largest organ, the liver, is a three-pound dynamo involved in most of the millions of physiological processes in the body and known to carry out more than five hundred functions. Probably the best-known function of the liver is detoxification, but it has many other important roles. There is something that you can do to help your liver out and detox the rest of "it."

Scott: What is "your body?"

Seymour: Way to go man! On a roll!

Scott: Yeah, now if I could just stop eating these donuts...

Howie: The liver is the workhorse of the body....Now no matter how dumb we act in regard to putting toxins in (environmental, dietary, etc.), it is smarter and will try to limit the continuous interaction with the already weakened immune system and insulate them in fat.

Scott: So, you're saying I can keep eating donuts, and the liver will sort it out?

Seymour: Well, not exactly. He said there was something you could do to help your liver out but thankfully, God did give us this amazing gift!

Scott: Donuts?

Seymour: (Shoots Scott a puzzled look)

Scott: I'm kidding.

500- Think of "it" as a nutritional bank. By making sufficient deposits, many transactions may be carried out each day.

Seymour: The banking system is so corrupt!

Host: Wrong book.

Scott: What is "my body?"

Host: YES!

Scott: And I promise I'm going to start viewing it like that and nourishing it with better food. I'm going to switch to jelly donuts since there's fruit in jelly, right?

Seymour: You're kidding right?

Sophia: I think he is but if not, remember, it's a process. Let's keep asking the right questions and thinking about the "end game."

Howie: Our bodies are equipped with the ability to repair themselves given that the equipment (our organs) have the integrity to function and have not been damaged beyond that point. *Moringa oleifera* definitely intervenes in this process offering the body the ability to heal itself.

THE PREVENTION IS THE CURE or AN OUNCE OF PREVENTION:

100- So it is sort of official….we can no longer take the approach of treating cancer…instead we should try this.

Seymour: Treating cancer is big business! Follow the money!

Host: Oh, sorry.

Seymour: Sorry, hard to resist.

Sophia: What is "an ounce of prevention?"

200- A new study shows that research to delay aging and the infirmities of old age would have better population health and economic returns than advances in individual fatal diseases.

Seymour: Who needs a study?

Host: No.

Scott: What is "the prevention is the cure?"

300- Get your nutrition from a safe source…raw, organic, vegan, enzymatically-alive nutrient rich and try to minimize the foods that damage you.

Seymour: That's what I'm talking about! I've been doing that for years! It's not easy or cheap. I spend a small fortune at the health food store!

Host: Well, that's too bad and incorrect.

Sophia: What is "an ounce of prevention?"

Scott: Yeah, think how much more that would cost you if you were paying British pounds! Good thing we whipped those Redcoats!

Seymour: Scott, you do realize…

Host: Save it for after the show.

400- Since even before the changes to the health care system, 80% of healthcare costs occur in the last ninety days of life, maybe we should consider this option…

Scott: What is getting rid of Obamacare!

Seymour: Or the Federal Reserve!

Host: No, sorry.

Sophia: What is "an ounce of prevention?"

Howie: This responsibility never eluded me since I have always sought the best when it comes to health in all aspects: nutrition, exercise, meditation, water quality, air purification, and radiation protection. As most of you will quickly have to adjust your thinking about health care, I suggest that you accept the responsibility for your health and be proactive.

500- It's worth a pound of cure!

Scott, Sophia, and Seymour in unison: What is "an ounce of prevention?"

Host: By George, I think you have all got it! I think this would be a good time for an interjection from Howie before our last category.

Howie: You cannot make someone listen although you know the value of an action. *Moringa oleifera* is that 'multi-million dollar penny' in the health arena. The value of retaining one's health and protecting yourself from free radical and inflammatory attacks on your body prevalent in our environment is more valuable than that 'penny.' Give your body what it needs, and your body will make its best effort to restore homeostasis.

It is always appreciated when a group such as the PHYSICIANS COMMITTEE FOR RESPONSIBLE MEDICINE contributes a quote that captures the essence of many of our nutritional deficits. Thanks for this wonderful quote.

"Sometimes the most elegant solution is the most simple. Why plant-based nutrition? Why not? Why develop heart disease? Cancer? Diabetes? The epidemic of chronic, degenerative disease that is sweeping the western world can not only be stopped; it can be reversed. The power lies in the hands of the consumer, in the choices we make about what to put on our plates."

MORINGA OLEIFERA:

100- In response to the dire situation whereby nutrition has been virtually eliminated from our diets "it" is the obvious solution.

Howie: It is more than 30% protein and therefore an extremely effective source of protein nutrition.

Seymour: What is "Moringa Oleifera?"

200- Its primary function is to repair and protect the liver everything else is simply a side-effect.

Scott: What is "Moringa Oleifera?"

Howie: It elevates glutathione levels to the extent that the glutathione levels protect the liver. Whoa....think about this. How much more does *Moringa oleifera* give than the significant elevation of glutathione levels?

300- *It* contains copious amounts of minerals such as zinc, calcium, iron, magnesium, copper, and many more. Each of these plays a unique physiological role in our health.

Sophia: What is "Moringa Oleifera?"

400- *This* tree aka the horseradish tree, drumstick tree, benzolive tree, kelor, marango, mlonge, moonga, mulangay, nébéday, saijhan, sajna or Ben oil tree (over 200 names), has been used by the ancient Hebrews, (Moses as directed by the Creator) Romans, Greeks and Egyptians.

Scott: What is "Moringa Oleifera?"

500- *A* tree native to India and the Himalayas but now cultivated in South America and Africa, it has been an important food source in some communities for millennia. The tree leaves pack a serious nutritional punch—we're talking high levels of 90 different nutrients, including protein, fiber, calcium, potassium, iron, vitamin C, and vitamin A. But, it's the plant's antioxidant content that has scientists really excited: 46 different kinds, to be exact.

All in unison: WHAT IS "MORINGA OLEIFERA?"

Host: So now it's time for...

FINAL..."This ain't Jeopardy."

However, it's been shown that our health is in danger which leads us to a most serious question. What, if anything can we do about it? Well, clearly we've seen that the prevention really is the cure and there are lots of preventive measures we can take. However, those measures aren't the focus of this book. That leads us to the Final "This Ain't Jeopardy" category which is...*Moringa Oleifera*

We have a rule here in "This Ain't Jeopardy" that all contestants will get to compete in Final This Ain't Jeopardy even if they finished the game in the negative. Why? Because much more is at stake here than money. This really is your life...no gameshow pun intended. So that's good news for Seymour and Scott, but we have another rule that is great for YOU, the reader. You get to make a wager too! We're all contestants in the game of health, and we must daily wager and ask the question, what's the value of this action? How much is your health worth?

Contestants, please make your wagers. We'll be back in a moment to see what the final answer is.

Host: Ok, we're back and the final "This Ain't Jeopardy" answer is...
"This mother of all adaptogens, this "miracle tree," this gift from a loving Creator, contains all of the following:

Amino Acids- Alanine, Arginine, Aspartic Acid, Cystine, Glutamine, Glutamic Acid, Glycine, Histidine, Isoleucine, Leucine, Lysine, Methionine, Phenylalanine, Proline, Serine, Threonine, Tryptophan, Tyrosine, Valine

Anti-Inflammatories- Arginine, Beta-sitosterol, Caffeoylquinic Acid, Calcium, Chlorophyll, Copper, Cystine, Omega 3, Omega 6, Omega 9, Fiber, Glutathione, Histidine, Indole Acetic Acid, Indoacetonitrile, Isoleucine, Kaempferal, Leucine, Magnesium, Oleic Acid, Phenylalanine, Potassium, Quercitin, Rutin, Selenium, Stigmasterol, Sulfur, Superoxide Dismutase, Tryptophan, Tyrosine, A, Thiamin (B1), C Ascorbic Acid, E Alpha Tocopherol, E (Delta Tocopherol), Zeatin, Zinc

Antioxidants- Alanine, Alpha-Carotene, Arginine, Beta-Carotene, Beta-sitosterol, Caffeoylquinic Acid, Campesterol, Carotenoids, Chlorophyll, Cholesterol, Chromium, Delta 5-Avenasterol, Glutathione, Histadine, Indole Acetic Acid, Indoleacetonitrile, Kaempferal, Lutein, Methionine, Myristic Acid, Palmitic Acid, Prolamine, Proline, Quercitin, Rutin, Selenium, Superoxide Dismutase, Threonine, Trytophan, A, B Choline, B1 Thiamin, B2 Riboflavin, B3 Niacin, B6 Pyroxidine, C Ascorbic Acid, E Alpha Tocopherol, E Delta Tocopherol, E Gamma Tocopherol, K, Xanthins, Xanthophyll, Zeatin, Zeaxanthin, Zinc, Carot- Alpha-Carotene, Beta-Carotene,

Chlorophyll, Lutein, Neoxanthin, Violaxanthin, Xanthophyll, Zeaxanthin

Cox 2-Inhibitors- Caffeoylquinic Acid, Kaempferol, Quercitin, Omega 3

Nutrients- Omega 3, Omega 6, Omega 9, Fiber, Flavenoids, Folate, Glutamine, Glutamic Acid, Iodine, Iron, Isoleucine, Leucine, Lutein, Lysine, Magnesium, Manganese, Methionine, Molybdenum, Phenylalanine, Phosphorus, Potassium, Protein, Threonine, Tryptophan, Valine, A, B Cholinbe, B1 Thiamin, B2 Riboflavin, B3 Niacin, B6 Pyroxidine, B12, C Ascorbic Acid, D, E, Zeaxanthin, Zinc, E Alpha Tocopherol

Fatty Acids- Arachidic Acid, Bechenic Acid, Gadoleic Acid, Lignoceric Acid, Myristic Acid, Omega 3, Omega 6, Omega 9, Palmitic Acid, Palmitoleic Acid, Stearic Acid, Kaempferol, Quercitin, Selenium

Glycosides- 4-Alpha-L-Rhamnosyloxy-Benzylglucosinate, 4-Alpha-L-Rhamnosyloxy-Senzylisothiocynate, Niazinin A, Niazinin B, Niaziminin A, Niaziminin B, Niazimicin, Rutin

Sterols- 28 Isoavenasterol, Betsitosterol, Brassicasterol, Campestanol, Campesterol, Cholesterol, Clerosterol, Delta-5-Avenasterol, Delta 7, 14 Stigmastanol, Delta 7 Avenasterol, Ergostadienol, Stigmastanol, Stigmasterol

Minerals- Calcium, Chromium, Cobalt, Copper, Fluorine, Iron, Lithium, Manganese, Magnesium, Molybdenum, Phosphorus, Potassium, Selenium, Silicon, Sodium, Sulfur, Vanadium, Zinc, Zirconium

Phenols- Caffeoylquinic Acid, Alpha Carotene, Beta Carotene, A, D, E Alpha Tocopherol, E Delta Tocopherol, E Gamma Tocopherol, K, Biotin. B1 Thiamin, B2 Riboflavin, B3 Niacin, B6 Pyridoxine,

C Ascorbic acid, Folate."
Host: While the contestants think, please enjoy our "This Ain't Jeopardy" theme music…

"A spoonful of raw, organic cane sugar helps the Moringa go down…"

…Ok, now it's time to see who is our winner today on "This Ain't Jeopardy."

We will now reveal our contestants' wagers and answers. I noticed Howie was slipping in Beatles song titles earlier so since we are short on time, I'm going to expedite things with one more.

"ALL TOGETHER NOW…" contestants…

Contestants: We wager it all….What is Moringa Oleifera?

Please visit us at http://moringadoctor.com/

Are you ready for a health revolution?:

Narrator: But wait, there's more. I told you there was a monster at the end of this book...

Gary: (In a mocking tone) You mean the guy in the kilt?

Dr. Howard W. Fisher

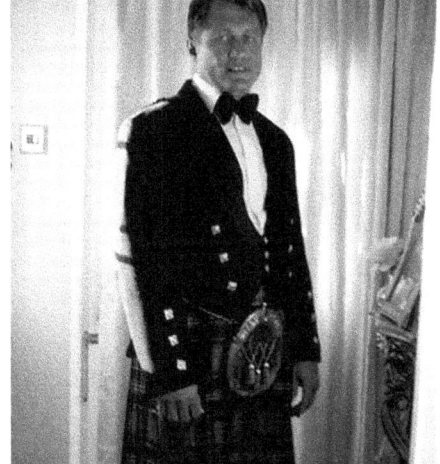

Narrator: William Wallace wore a kilt.

Gary: That's William Wallace? I thought William Wallace was taller.

Narrator: No, that's not William Wallace. Though, in my humble opinion, he is doing far more to advance the cause of freedom for far more people. He is a crusader for health freedom. Now, he invites you to join our army. Moringa is our weapon of choice. With it, we plan to ignite a "health revolution" and paradigm-shift in the way our communities look at healthcare from a system of disease management to one of wellness and disease prevention.

Gary: Well, if it's not William Wallace, why is he wearing a kilt?

Narrator: If you're not a rat, why are you letting them prescribe you rat poison and other chemicals to exterminate you?

Gary: Who is "them"?

Howie: Careful…let them come to their own conclusions… share don't push.

Narrator: If William Wallace were here today, what do you think he would say to those people that are conspiring to kill us?

Gary: He wouldn't have to say or do anything. If such people existed, I would kill them myself.

Howie: Easy. Anyone can fight but like my older brother Bobby taught us, "it's our wits that make us men."

Narrator: (Fact check) It's Bobby Fischer with a "c" and that quote is from *Braveheart*.

Howie: Well, I didn't say it. In fact, I'm not even really here right now—only a figment of your runaway imagination.

Narrator: But that really is you wearing a kilt in that picture?

Howie: Yes.

Narrator: You are a health freedom advocate and the author of 20 books on health?

Howie: Correct.

Seymour: He's a patriot!

Narrator: Yet, like William Wallace, there are some in the "medical mafia" who might call him a traitor and seek to…

William Wallace: I am William Wallace!

Gary: Is this a dream?

William Wallace: No, it's the imaginative portion of a book about Moringa.

Gary: I really thought William Wallace was taller and would have a sword.

William Wallace: I have a much better weapon than a sword.

Gary: What's that?

William Wallace: I have in my possession the most phytonutrient plant ever discovered.

Gary: Not sure you'll be able to kill many enemies with that.

William Wallace: I'm not here to kill but to heal. This is a plant given by our Almighty Creator to nourish and enable the body to restore itself as He intended.

Gary: Is it Scottish?

William Wallace: No.

Gary: If it's not Scottish...

William Wallace: Are you Scottish?

Gary: No.

Scott: Is it American?

William Wallace: No.

Scott: Russian?

William Wallace: Nyet.

Scott: French?

William Wallace: *bien sûr que non... (of course not)*

Gary: Wait, this is my dream—I'll ask the questions.

William Wallace: This is my army and to join it you must answer 15 questions.

Gary: Why 15 and who said I wanted to join your army?

William Wallace: Well, it's 15 questions because we are playing a game called, "Who wants to be a Moringa-naire?

Gary: Is that even a real game?

William Wallace: It is now.

Gary: Why?

William Wallace: "I AM WILLIAM WALLACE! And I see a whole host of my fellow countrymen here in defiance of worse than any tyranny than I ever fought in Scotland! They are trying to make you a slave, man! Stand up and fight! Fight with your intellect! Fight with your right to make your own decisions about your own health! Do it, and you may live. Do it not…

Gary: I thought you said, "every man dies…"

William Wallace: Yes, but "not every man truly lives."

Gary: But my doctors have promised me a 5 % chance if I take their…

William Wallace: STOP! Listen to yourself. You are clinging to some meager percentage given you by fallible doctors instead of taking responsibility for your own actions and health and just trusting God to preserve you with what he is given to sustain your fearfully and wonderfully made body! That's worse than "squabbling for scraps from Longshanks table!" You truly do have a God-given right to plants! And I'm offering you the best plant ever discovered! Did you not listen to that man wearing the kilt?

Gary: It's hard to trust a doctor wearing a kilt.

William Wallace: You prefer a lab coat? As another doctor might say, "How's that working for ya?"

Gary: Dr. Phil?

Narrator: No, he's not here, but Howie does a great impersonation during his lectures.

Gary: Howie?

Narrator: Dr. Fisher. The guy in the kilt. Try to keep up. Your life is in jeopardy.

Gary: Ok. I admit things haven't been working really well.

William Wallace: You ready to try another way?

Gary: It's much to risk. I could die.

William Wallace: Again, every man dies. I promise you not eternal life. Only God may grant you that. But that same God has given you "every herb bearing seed, which *is* upon the face of all the earth, and every tree, in which *is* the fruit of a tree yielding seed; to you, it shall be for meat." Do you trust Him?

Gary: I want to believe.

William Wallace: He's ready. Let the game begin.

Host: Welcome back folks! It's time for "Who wants to be a health-o-naire?"

Howie: Not specific enough. Narrow the focus. Remember, we seek simple and BEST.

CHAPTER 13

Who wants to be a ~~"Health-o-naire?"~~ Moringa-naire?

Host: Are you ready to play?

Gary: Me?

Host: Yes, are you ready to play, "Who wants to be a "health-o-naire?"

Howie: Moringa...

Host: Oh yeah, I know Doc.

Howie: If you know, why do you keep saying it?

Host: Well, I've just gotten so used to seeing people who take Moringa get healthy, it's hard not to see them as one and the same.

Howie: The impossible takes about 120 days, miracles slightly longer...

Scott: Like the "Miracle on Ice?"

Seymour: That wasn't a miracle. The Russians actually threw the game to...

Host: Guys, let's not get off on other tangents or conspiracy theories. However, I agree the word "miracle" gets thrown around way too much. In fact, when you really think about it, it's not even a miracle if you get a good result from a plant God created and gave to man as a gift for health. It would actually just be the logical consequence of following God's prescription for health. Of course, God can heal miraculously if He chose to and certainly there are plenty of examples of that in the Bible but generally, He uses means. And what better means to a healthy end than the most nutrient dense plant God ever created!

Howie: You're right. Lots of people begin seeing results immediately as this is such a potent plant, but I'm referring to the life cycle of red blood cells. And this is why you need to go on a course of *Moringa oleifera* for at least 120 days or, like the smart people, for the rest of your life.

Host: Great, without further ado, let's see who really wants to be a Moringa-naire for the rest of their life!

Host: So let's go over the rules. As always, whether you're Gary who is playing here on the "live show" or you're one of the readers at home, we insist on keeping it simple for our contestants. Regardless of whether you're facing a serious health challenge or you just want to make daily incremental progress towards better health, it's always BEST to keep it simple. Whether it's on the chess board or...

Howie: Are you going to use another chess analogy?

Host: You guessed it.

Howie: Ok, whatever keeps it simple for you and the reader.

Host: There is a poignant scene in the movie, *Searching for Bobby Fischer* where the young chess prodigy, Josh Waitzkin and his coach, Bruce Pandolfini, are sitting across from each other at a chessboard looking over a position.
"Mate is 4 moves from the position in front of you," says the coach played by actor Ben Kingsley. With confidence and clarity, he continues, "Don't move until you figure it out in your head. Don't look to me for a hint."
An exasperated Waitzkin responds, "I can't do it without moving the pieces." His coach remains resolute exhorting him further, "Yes you can. Clear the lines of men in your head, one at a time and the king will be left standing alone, like a guy on a street corner."
At that point, the coach looks at Josh and says, "…Here, I'll make it easier for you…" and simultaneously sweeps the pieces off of the board onto the floor with the back of his right hand and forearm. With the camera focused on the blank board, the coach says to Josh, "…Now you can solve it…"[346]

Gary: I'm confused. Are we playing chess or "Who wants to be a Moringa-naire?"

Host: Neither and both.

Gary: Huh?

Host: We are playing the game of life and remember that "life is a kind of chess," and in the game we are playing today, we will ask questions that have the potential to greatly change the trajectory of your life. Believe it or not, there is a clear solution for you, Gary. There's also a clear solution to the issues we have brought up in this book regarding the poor quality of health and nutrition we face today, especially in North America. However, it's only when we "clear the lines in our head" that we can engage in the deep thinking necessary to solve such problems.

Therefore, I challenge you Gary, and you, reader, to "clear the lines…in your head, one at a time" until the solution becomes obvious. Don't move until you see it. You may, however, look to me for a hint. You may also look back in the book, poll the audience, ask or phone a friend on any question. That's right—unlimited lifelines!

If you still need help, you may also visit http://moringadoctor.com/ and who knows—maybe you can even speak to the Doc himself!

Because this is a game with very serious consequences. If you make a mistake on a chess board, no big deal—you simply lose a game. You make a mistake in this "kind of chess," it can actually cost you your life.

Therefore, it is imperative we come up with a clear winning strategy. I've heard commentators use the phrase, "conceptual chess" referring to theoretical ideas a grandmaster may have which he must back up with concrete moves at the board. He must prove his strategy was sound. Here, we are doing the same thing—call it "conceptual health" if you will. Remember the Crocodile Dundee illustration Howie used? We really do insist that Moringa is "that knife" in the nutrient world and we plan to wield it with precision to save lives and enhance the health of "our neighbors."

Gary: But isn't it too late for theories now? I'm dying.

Host: We're all going to die.

Gary: But I have terminal cancer. They said I have less than a year to live.

Host: Who told you that?! Don't answer that—it doesn't matter. Nobody has the right to tell you that! They aren't God!

Gary: But they are the doctors. They have done tests. They are experts.

Host: And yet, these experts don't know or care how you got this "cancer" and gave you no real solution. Sounds like intellectual lazy thinking at best and...

Howie: Let him come to his own conclusions...

Host: Ok, Gary, so you arrived here today in a tough position. You're sitting there thinking I'm two moves away from being checkmated. You feel defeated. It is a terribly demoralizing situation but believe it or not, there is hope. The good news is you are still alive, and the better news is that there is an omnipotent God who may yet heal you in any number of ways He may choose.

Gary: Well, I'm still in the game I guess…I might as well keep playing.

Host: Great. Let's play. Let's look for a clear strategy—let's find a path to victory, a winning combination.

Gary: I hope so, but I confess I ain't the sharpest knife in the drawer.

Host: Well, don't worry, Gary. "This ain't Jeopardy." Sorry, I couldn't resist. And I ain't that smart myself, but I do have access to the greatest lifeline of all, and so do you—an all-knowing God who we may go to for wisdom. (James 1:5-8).

WHO WANTS TO BE A MORINGA-NAIRE? (Easy-peasy version)

Host: Ok, so this shouldn't be a very difficult quiz for most of you whether or not you read the book. The "monster" will come after the test as again we try to lead you in a logical order to a "precise move." If you have any trouble answering, feel free to use a lifeline. So here we go…with no commercial interruptions and limited interjections.

As in "This Ain't Jeopardy," we start with…

PROBLEMS

1. The food chain is…
   A. Broken B. Nutrient-deficient C. Lacking minerals D. All of the above

2. Indications of a Vitamin C deficiency include:
   A. weakness B. fatigue C. bruising easily and increased healing time D. All of the above

3. Indications of a Vitamin B-12 deficiency include:
   A. mental fatigue and poor concentration B. poor circulation C. decreased REM sleep D. All of the above

4. Indications of a Vitamin D deficiency include:
   A. poor blood sugar stability B. chronic pain C. gait and clumsiness issues D. All of the above

5. Indications of a Magnesium deficiency include:
   A. constipation/irregular bowel activity B. indigestion C. decreased enzymatic activity (zinc is also very important here) D. All of the above

6. Indications of an Omega Essential Fatty Acids deficiency include:
   A. depression B. hormone imbalance C. neurological problems, D. All of the above

Host: Ok, it's going to get slightly harder as we throw out the "all of the above" answers. Don't worry, we will provide some hints.

SOLUTIONS

7. According to Professor Helena Baranova, 85%-96% of disease is due to _____.
   A. your shoe size B. environmental factors C. your favorite color D. your inherited genes

Howie: I always have been a proponent that our lifestyle choices can move us from the chronological clock to a physiological clock.

8. So it is sort of official....we can no longer take the approach of treating cancer...we have to do this to build health.
   A. get preventive B. go to the moon C. beat the Russians in hockey D. watch more TV

Seymour: You would think if we could actually go to the moon, then we could also figure out how to prevent and reverse disease...

Host: Ok, that is officially the last conspiracy theory you get to mention.

Howie: I have been on this preventive approach for thirty years, and now they realize the importance of diet and environment. I think perhaps the introduction of a phytonutrient dense plant would be the perfect intervention.

9. In 1958, two Russian doctors, I.I. Brekhman and I.V. Dardymov defined _____: "A substance that is innocuous and cause minimal disorders in the physiological functions of an organism, it must have a nonspecific action, and it usually has a normalizing action irrespective of the direction of the pathological state." The bottom line translation of this is give your body what it needs, and your body will respond.
A. chemotherapy B. radiation C. an adaptogen D. kryptonite

Seymour: So we claim to have beat them in the space race, hockey, and the cold war but they figured out adaptogens long before any of it?

Host: You just gave away the answer and uttered another conspiracy theory. I must ask you to leave the studio.

10. Which of the following is NOT an example of a plant made by God?
A. chlorella B. broccoli C. Moringa oleifera D. donuts

11. Of the aforementioned plants, this one has more of chlorophyll, protein, iron, vitamins, and minerals and a lot more antioxidants, Omega 3 FAs, chlorophyll,

anti-inflammatory phytonutrients...well, in fact, pretty much everything you need...
A. Moringa oleifera B. chlorella C. broccoli D. donuts

12. The leaves of *"this"* extraordinary tree contain seven times the vitamin C found in oranges, seventeen times the calcium in milk, ten times the vitamin A in carrots, nine times the protein of yogurt, twenty-five times the iron in spinach, three times the vitamin E of almonds, and fifteen times the potassium in bananas.
A. apple tree B. Moringa oleifera C. family tree D. donut tree

13. In addition to its many known benefits, there is evidence that Moringa oleifera has the potential to do all of the following except...
A. potential to kill bacteria and parasites B. fight diabetes C. reduce inflammation throughout the body D. Helps pigs fly

Gary: It sure sounds good enough to make pigs fly. And I've already been told there is no cure for diabetes. So I choose B.

Host: Is that your final answer?

Howie: My interest in Moringa stems from the knowledge that poor nutrition has been linked to the major chronic diseases, immune system dysfunction and premature aging that are affecting the global population leading to a decreased quality of life. *Moringa* delivers nutrition that has systematically been removed from the food chain.

Gary: Ok, on second thought, I choose D.

14. Thomas Edison is quoted as saying, "The doctor of the future will no longer give medicine," but rather:
   A. prescribe 6-8 hours of TV each day B. instruct his patient in the care of the human frame, in diet, and in the cause and prevention of disease C. recommend more processed/fast food D. give out lollipops

Host: It's a great quote, but it's not in the book so we will give you 50/50 and take away two of the choices. You are left with B and C.

Gary: Good thing cause my doctor does pass out lollipops and all kinds of candy. I'll choose B.

Host: Correct! Now for the final question.

15. It has already been demonstrated that no agency will safeguard your health better than ____.
   A. The CDC B. The AMA C. Homeland Security D. You

So, is it time for YOU to become your own "doctor of the future" by prescribing Moringa oleifera for yourself?

BONUS: IF you answered a resounding YES...

16. When looking for the BEST source of Moringa oleifera, you should make sure it is...
   A. Organically-grown B. Hand-picked C. Shade-dried D. All of the above

Dr. Howard W. Fisher & Steve Wilson

THE MONSTER AT THE END OF THE BOOK

No, it's not the guy in the kilt. It's not loveable furry old Grover either. It's you. It's up to you to go beyond the three R's you learned in school. I recently interviewed one of America's premier Grand Masters, Yasser Seirawan for a "Chess Matters" book (coming soon) and he told me chess teaches the 5 R's; reading, writing, arithmetic, reasoning, and responsibility.

Reading: You've read the book. You can feel free to check out the end notes and read more on Moringa.

Writing: Write your answers to the questions above or write an advantages/disadvantages list of taking Moringa oleifera. For example…

Advantages	Disadvantages
• More chlorophyll, protein, iron, vitamins, and minerals and a lot more antioxidants, Omega 3 FAs, chlorophyll, anti-inflammatory phytonutrients…well, in fact, pretty much everything you need. • Contains seven times the vitamin C found in oranges. • Contains seventeen times the calcium in milk. • Contains ten times the vitamin A in carrots. • Contains nine times the protein of yogurt. • Contains twenty-five times the iron in spinach. • Contains fifteen times the potassium in bananas. • May help pigs fly??	• Cost ?? • Discipline to take it daily.

Arithmetic: Remember the statistic that 80% of healthcare costs occur in the last ninety days of life. Remember that your health really is your wealth. What's it worth? What's the true value of an action like finding that "multi-million dollar penny in the health arena?" Figure out what it would cost you to take Moringa on a daily basis and find a way to fit it in your budget.

Reasoning: Clear the lines in your head. Think deeply. Does this make sense? What is the best move?

"It's almost all theory and memorization. People think there are all these options, but there's usually one right move..."—Bobby Fischer as quoted in *Pawn Sacrifice.*

While I personally wouldn't want to take Bobby Fischer's end game advice in the game of life, I love the quote above. To me, it encompasses much more than what might happen in a complex and yet simple game. Yes, chess, like life, like one's health might be hard to make sense of for us mortals. Or, it could be much simpler than we make it out to be. What if there really is an omnipotent God who made me and gives me a theory and facts to memorize (in His Word) which may actually lead me to a thought which enables me to make that "one right move?" That's my "theory of everything" and I'm sticking to it.

So what's your theory? What have you memorized? How do you know it's the right theory? What's your objective standard of truth? Can you back it up with concrete moves? Do you have an end game?

There are many good moves to be made in this life. There are many good moves for health. There are even many good moves for nutrition. Yet, that's not why we put forth this book. We asked one very important question in the beginning of this book which we now ask YOU to answer.

Is there a plant given by a loving and wise Creator which is able to replace the missing amino acid profiles and supply an enzymatically active, bioavailable, antioxidant-rich, anti-inflammatory rich, natural source of nutrition?

OR perhaps even simpler: Is there a nutritional BEST bang for the buck for the whole living, breathing, dying world?

The authors have made their choice. You've read the testimonials of many others who have chosen Moringa oleifera as their "nutritional best." But what say YOU? If you agree with us, read the next paragraph. If not, I invite you to my health island any time to tell me why you disagree. Perhaps we can play a healthy game of chess and discuss it.

Responsibility: Well, if you are here, you have made it to the real "monster at the end of this book." Taking Responsibility is our last "R" but certainly not least. This one can be a real beast. In the end, you're the "chess player" and you must take responsibility for the moves you make as well as the moves you should make but don't. It's one thing to believe "this move works" but it's a far different thing to actually pick the piece up and set it down on another square. However, for change to come, this is exactly what you must do. I know it's hard especially when you are being bombarded with opinions from everywhere. I know there are "those people" out there jerking on you every moment with scare tactics and gloom and doom statistics telling you that you are going to die if you don't "do what we say." It's worse than SAD…it's downright despicable.

Well, as Howie often says, "we share, don't push." We offer hope, not scare or manipulation tactics. I'll use one last metaphor but this time it's not chess. Let's think of our health as a "kind of ship" which sometimes must sail through troubled waters. There is a storm raging and the ship is in danger of sinking. Don't worry though. You know what must be done. There's a simple solution. It's time to throw the "jetsam" overboard before you are sunk. Do whatever it takes to keep only what is necessary on board your "health ship." Or maybe it's time to abandon ship!

Gary: I thought you said no scare tactics?

Narrator: I'm not. I'm inviting them on our *Moringa Matters* cruise ship.

Gary: Let me guess…"where you sail a sea of green…every one of you has all you need?"

Narrator: No, not a Yellow Submarine…but that does give me an idea…

Howie: Save it for another book.

BIBLIOGRAPHY

1. Baranova H. **New Look on Anti-Ageing Medicine through Genomics and Evidence Based Medicine. What Can Be Done In Practice.** 4th Annual Anti-Ageing Conference London 2007 (AACL) The Royal Society of Medicine. **September 16, 2007.**
2. U.S. Department of Health and Human Service Centers for Disease Control and Prevention. National Center for Health Statistics. Deaths – Leading Causes 2009. http://www.cdc.gov/nchs/fastats/lcod.htm.
3. Giovannucci E, Stampfer M J, Colditz G A, Hunter D J, Fuchs C, et al. Multivitamin use, folate and colon cancer in women in the Nurses' Health Study. *Ann Intern Med.* 1998; 129(7):p517-24.
4. Giovannucci E, Ascherio A, Rimm E B, Stampfer M J, Colditz G A, Willett W. Intake of carotenoids and retinol in relation to risk of prostate cancer. *J Natl Cancer Inst.* 1995; 87: p1767-1776.
5. NIH Record. NIH Celebrates Earth Day 2008. Vol LX. No.6. March 21, 2008. http://nihrecord.od.nih.gov/newsletters/2008/03_21_2008/story4.htm
6. Feher J, Csomos G, Verekei A. Free radical reactions in medicine. 1st Ed. Germany. Springer Verlag. 1987;p.11.
7. Southorn P A. Free radicals in medicine I. Chemical nature and biologic reactions. *Mayo Clinic Proc.* 1988;63:p.381-389.

8. Baynes J W. Role of oxidative stress in development and complications in diabetes. *Diabetes.* 1991;40:p.405-412.
9. Sinclair A J. Free radical mechanism and vascular complication of diabetes mellitus. *Diabetes Rev.* 1993;2:p.7-11.
10. Giugliano D, Ceriello A, Paoliso G. Oxidative stress and diabetic complications. *Diabet Care.* 1996;19:p.257-267.
11. Mullenix PS, Andersen CA, Starnes BW. Atherosclerosis as inflammation. *Ann Vasc Surg.*2005;19:p.130–138.
12. Libby P, Theroux P. Pathophysiology of coronary artery disease. *Circulation.* 2005;111:p.3481–3488.
13. Hansson GK. Inflammation, atherosclerosis, and coronary artery disease. *N Engl J Med.*2005;352:1685–1695.
14. Sun Y, Campisi J, Higano C, Beer T M, Porter P, Coleman I, True L, Nelson P S. Treatment-induced damage to the tumor microenvironment promotes prostate cancer therapy resistance through WNT16B. *Nature Medicine* 2012; 18:p.1359-1368.
15. Sreelatha S, Padma P R. Antioxidant activity and total phenolic content of Moringa oleifera leaves in two stages of maturity. Plant Foods Hum Nutr. 2009;64:p.303–311.
16. Moyo B, Masika P J, Hugo A, Muchenje V. Nutritional characterization of Moringa (*Moringa oleifera* **Lam.) leaves.** *African Journal of Biotechnology.* 2011; October 5. Vol.10 (60), p. 12925-12933.
17. Zamora-Ros R, Rothwell J A, Scalbert A, Knaze V, Romieu I, Slimani N, Fagherazzi G, Perquier F, Touillaud M, Molina-Montes E, Huerta J M, Barricarte A, Amiano P, Menendez V, Tumino R, Santucci de Magis M, Palli D, Ricceri F, Sieri S. Crowe F L, Khaw K T, Wareham N J, Grote V, Li K, Boeing H, Foerster J, Trichopoulou A, Benetou V, Tsiotas K, Bueno-de-Mesquita, Ros M, Peeters P H M, Tjonneland A, Halkjaer J, Overvad K, Ericson U, Wallström P, Johansson I, Landberg R, Weiderpass E, Engeset D, Skeie G, Wark P, Riboli E, Gonzalez C A. Dietary intakes and food sources of phenolic acids in the European Prospective Investigation into Cancer and Nutrition (EPIC) study. *B J Nutr.* 2013;110(8):p.1500-1511.

18. Bennett R N, Mellon F A, Foidl N, Pratt J H, Dupont M S, Perkins L, Kroon P A. Profiling glucosinolates and phenolics in vegetative and reproductive tissues of the multi-purpose trees Moringa oleifera L. (horseradish tree) and Moringa stenopetala L. J Agric Food Chem. 2003;51:p.3546–3553.
19. Arisi MF, Starker RA, Addya S, Huang Y, Fernandez SV. All trans-retinoic acid (ATRA) induces re-differentiation of early transformed breast epithelial cells. Int J Oncol. 2014; June 44(6):p.1831-1842.
20. Black R E, Allen L H, Bhutta Z A, Caulfield L E. Maternal and child undernutrition: global and regional exposures and health consequences, The Lancet, 2008, 371(9608), p. 253.
21. Marler J B, Wallin J R. Human Health, the Nutritional Quality of Harvested Food and Sustainable Farming Systems. Nutrition Security Insitute 2006
22. ibid
23. Ji Y, Tan S, Xu Y, Chandra A, Shi C, Song B, Qin J, Gao Y. Vitamin B supplementation, homocysteine levels, and the risk of cerebrovascular disease: A meta-analysis. *Neurology*. 2013, September 18.
24. ibid
25. Starobrat-Hermelin B, Kozielec T. The effects of magnesium physiological supplementation on hyperactivity in children with attention deficit hyperactivity disorder (ADHD). Positive response to magnesium oral loading test. *Magnes Res*. 1997; Jun;10(2):p.149-56
26. Dodig-Curković K, Dovhanj J, Curković M, Dodig-Radić J, Degmecić D. The role of zinc in the treatment of hyperactivity disorder in children. *Acta Med Croatica*. 2009 Oct;63(4):307-13. Review. Croatian.
27. Wong C P, Magnusson K R, Ho E. Increased inflammatory response in aged mice is associated with age-related zinc deficiency and zinc transporter dysregulation. J Nut Biochem. 2013;24(1):p353-359.
28. Wong C P, Magnusson K R, Ho E. Increased inflammatory response in aged mice is associated with age-related zinc deficiency and zinc transporter dysregulation. J Nut Biochem. 2013;24(1):p353-359.

29. Fakurazi S, Hairuszah I, Nanthini U. Moringa oleifera prevents acetaminophen induced liver injury through restoration of glutathione level. 2008. Food Chem. Toxicol. 46, p.2611–2615
30. Fakurazi S, Hairuszah I, Nanthini U. Moringa oleifera prevents acetaminophen induced liver injury through restoration of glutathione level. 2008. Food Chem. Toxicol. 46, p.2611–2615.
31. Yang R Y, Tsou S C S, Lee T C, Chang L C, Kuo G, Lai P Y. Moringa, a novel plant rich in antioxidants, bioavailable iron, and nutrients. In Wang M (ed), Herbs: Challenges in Chemistry and Biology of Herbs, Am. Chem. Soc. US 2006; p p224-239.
32. Sharma V, Paliwal R. Potential Chemoprevention of 7,12-Dimethylbenz[a]anthracene Induced Renal Carcinogenesis by Moringa oleifera Pods and Its Isolated Saponin. Indian J Clin Biochem. 2014 Apr;29(2):202-9
33. Baranov A S, Chernova O F, Feoktistova N Y, Surov A V, "A New Example of Ectopia: Oral Hair in Some Rodent Species," Doklady Biological Sciences, 2010, Vol. 431, p. 117–120, Original Russian Text © A.S. Baranov, O.F. Chernova, N.Yu. Feoktistova, A.V. Surov, 2010, published in Doklady Akademii Nauk, 2010, Vol. 431, No. 4, pp. 559–562.
34. Friel J P, ed. Dorland's Illustrated Medical Dictionary. Twenty-fifth Edition. W.B. Saunders. Philadelphia. 1974.
35. Gunderson E L. *FDA Total Diet Survey, April 1982-April 1986, Dietary intakes of pesticides, selected elements and other chemicals.* Food and Drug Administration, Division of Contaminants Chemistry. Washington, DC 20204.
36. Houlihan J, Kropp T, Wiles R, Gray S, Campbell C. Body burden—the pollution in newborns: A benchmark investigation of industrial chemicals, pollutants and pesticides in umbilical cord blood. Environmental Working Group. July 14, 2005.
37. Edwards T. Inflammation, pain, and chronic disease: an integrative approach to treatment and prevention. *Alter Ther Health Med.* 2005;Nov-Dec 11(6):p.20-27.

38. *Di Giuseppe D, Wallin A, Bottai M, Askling J, Wolk A.* Long-term intake of dietary long-chain n-3 polyunsaturated fatty acids and risk of rheumatoid arthritis: a prospective cohort study of women. *Ann Rheum Dis.* 2013 Aug 12
39. Rahman M M, Kopec J A, Anis A H, Cibere J, Goldsmith C H. "Risk of cardiovascular disease in patients with osteoarthritis: a prospective longitudinal study." Arthritis Care Res (Hoboken). 2013 Dec;65(12):p.1951-8.
40. Youm Y H, Grant R W, McCabe, L R., Albarado D C, Nguyen, K Y, Ravussin, A, Dixit A, Deep V et al. Canonical Nlrp3 Inflammasome Links Systemic Low-Grade Inflammation to Functional Decline in Aging. Cell metabolism, volume 18 issue 4 pp.519-532.
41. Cheng Y J, Hootman J M, Murphy L B, Langmaid G A, Helmick C G. Prevalence of doctor-diagnosed arthritis and arthritis-attributable activity limitation—United States, 2007–2009. *MMWR* 2010;59(39):p.1261–1265.
42. Hootman J M, Helmick C G. Projections of U.S. prevalence of arthritis and associated activity limitations. *Arthritis Rheum* 2006;54(1):p.266–229.
43. Berbert A A, Kondo C R, Almendra C L et al. Supplementation of fish oil and olive oil in patients with rheumatoid arthritis. *Nutrition.* 2005;21:p.131-136.
44. Hagen K B, Byfuglien MG, Falzon L, Olsen SU, Smedslund G. Dietary interventions for rheumatoid arthritis. *Cochrane Database Syst Rev.* 2009; Jan 21;(1):CD006400.
45. Kremer J M. N-3 fatty acid supplements in rheumatoid arthritis. *Am J Clin Nutr.* 2000;(suppl 1)p.349S-351S.
46. Ruggiero C, Lattanzio F, Lauretani F, et al. Omega-3 polyunsaturated fatty acids and immune-mediated dieases: inflammatory bowel disease and rheumatoid arthritis. *Curr Pharm Des.* 2009; 15(36): p.4135-4138.
47. Sales C, Oliviero F, Spinella P. The Mediterranean diet model in inflammatory rheumatic diseases. *Reumatismo.* 2009; 61(1): p.10-14.

48. Galarraga B, Ho M, Youssef H M, et al. Cod liver oil (n-3 fatty acids) as an non-steroidal anti-inflammatory drug sparing agent in rheumatoid arthritis. *Rheumatology* (Oxford) 2008;47(5):p.665-669.
49. Bahadori B, Uitz E, Thonhofer R, et al. omega-3 fatty acids infusions as adjuvant therapy in rheumatoid arthritis. *JPEN J Parenter Enteral Nutr.* 2010;34(2):p.151-5.
50. Curtis C L, Rees S G, Little C B, et al. Pathologic indicators of degradation and inflammation in human osteoarthritic cartilage are abrogated by exposure to n-3 fatty acids. *Arthritis Rheum.* 2002;46(6):p.1544-1553.
51. Zainal Z, Longman AJ, Hurst S, et al. Relative efficacies of omega-3 polyunsaturated fatty acids in reducing expression of key proteins in a model system for studying osteoarthritis. *Osteoarthritis Cartilage.* 2009;17(7):p.896-905.
52. Goldberg R J, Katz J. A meta-analysis of the analgesic effects of omega-3 polyunsaturated fatty acid supplementation for inflammatory joint pain. *Pain.* 2007; May 29⊛1-2):p.210-223.
53. Anhwange B A, Ajibola V O, Oniye S J. Chemical studies of the seeds of *Moringa oleifera*(Lam) and Detarium microcarpum (Guill and Sperr). *J Biological Sci.* 2004;4:p.711-715.
54. Paliwal **R, Sharma V, Pracheta V. A review on Horse Radiah Tree (*Moringa oleifera*): A Multipurpose Tree with High Economic and Commercial Importance. Asian Journal of Biotechnology. 2011;3(4):p.317-328.**
55. Fuglie L J. *The Miracle Tree: Moringa oleifera: Natural Nutrition for the Tropics.* Church World Service, Dakar. 1999:68pp.
56. Anwar F, Latif S, Ashraf M, Gilani A H. *Moringa oleifera*: A food plant with multiple medicinal uses. *Phytother Res.* 2007;21:p.17-25.
57. Delaveau P, et al. Oils of *Moringa oleifera* and Moringa drouhardii. *Plantes Médicinales et Phytothérapie.* 1980;14(10):p.29-33.
58. Caceres A, Saravia A, Rizzo S, Zabala L, Leon E D, Nave F. Pharmacological properties of *Moringa oleifera*. 2: Screening for antispasmodic, anti-inflammatory and diuretic activity. *J Ethnopharmacol.* 1992;36:p.233-237.

59. Ezeamuzie I C, Ambakederemo A W, Shode F O, Ekwebelm S C. Antiinflammatory effects of *Moringa oleifera* root extract. *Int J Pharmacog.* 1996;34(3):p.207-212.
60. Rao K N V, Gopalakrishnan V, Loganathan V, Shanmuganathan S. Antiinflammatory activity of *Moringa oleifera* Lam. *Ancient Science of Life.* 1999;18(3-4):p.195-198.
61. Udapa S L, Udapa A L, et al. Studies on the anti-inflammatory and wound healing properties of *Moringa oleifera* and Aegle marmelos. *Fitoterapia.* 1994;65(2):p.119-123.
62. Pari L, Kumar N A. Hepatoprotective activity of *Moringa oleifera* on antitubercular drug-induced liver damage in rats. *J Med Foods.* 2002;5(3): p.171-177.
63. Ibid
64. Buraimoh A A. Hepatoprotective effect of ethanolic leave extract of *Moringa oleifera* on the histology of paracetamol induced liver damage in Wistar rats. Int J Anim Vet Adv.2011;3:p.10-13.
65. Kelsey M M, Zaepfel A, Bjornstad P, Nadeau K J. Age-related consequences of childhood obesity. *Gerontology.* 2014;60(3):p.222-8. doi: 10.1159/000356023. Epub 2014 Jan 9
66. Holmes M V, Lange L A Palmer T.et al, "Causal Effects of Body Mass Index on Cardiometabolic Traits and Events: A Mendelian Randomization Analysis," The American Journal of Human Genetics, 2014;Volume 94, Issue 2, 6 February p.198-208.
67. Beach, R. Modern Miracle Men. US Senate Document 264. 1936.
68. Lustig R. Fat Chance: The bitter truth about sugar. Hudson Street Press, Penguin Group USA. 2013.
69. Ramachandran C, Peter K V, Gopalakrishnan P K. 1980, Drumstick (*Moringa oleifera*): A multipurpose Indian Vegetable. *Economic Botany*, 34 (3) p.276-283.
70. Rana J .S, Nieuwdorp M, Jukema J W, Kastelein J J. Cardiovascular metabolic syndrome – an interplay of, obesity, inflammation, diabetes and coronary heart disease. Diabetes Obes. Metab. 2007;9:p.218-232.

71. Wild S, Roglic G, Green A, Sicree R, King H. Global prevalence of diabetes: estimates for the year 2000 and projections for 2030. *Diabetes Care.* 2004:27:p.1047-1053.
72. Cousens G. *There Is a Cure for Diabetes.* North Atlantic Books. Berkeley California. 2008.
73. Dieye A M, Sarr A, Diop S N, Ndiaye M, Sy G Y, Diarra M, Rajraji Gaffary I, Ndiaye Sy A., Faye B. Medicinal plants and the treatment of diabetes in Senegal: survey with patients. *Fundam. Clin. Pharmacol.* 2008;22: p.211-216.
74. Ghiridhari V V A, Malhati D, Geetha K. Anti-diabetic properties of drumstick (*Moringa oleifera*) leaf tablets. Int. *J.HealthNutr.* 2011;2:p.1-5.
75. Jaiswal D, Kumar Rai P, Kumar A, Mehta S, Watal G. Effect of *Moringa oleifera* Lam. leaves aqueous extract therapy on hyperglycemic rats. *J Ethnopharmacol.* 2009;123:p.392-396.
76. Ndong M, Uehara M, Katsumata S, Suzuki K. Effects of oral administration of *Moringa oleifera* Lam on glucose tolerance in Goto-Kakizaki and Wistar rats. J. Clin. Biochem. Nutr. 2007b;40: p.233–229.
77. William F, Lakshminarayanan S, Chegu H. Effect of some Indian vegetables on the glucose and insulin response in diabetic subjects. *Int j Food Sci Nutr.* 1993;44:p.191-196.
78. Kumari D J. Hypoglycemic effect of *Moringa fera* and *Azadirachta indica* in type2- diabetes *Bioscan.* 2010;5:p.211-214
79. Cho A S, Jeon S M, Kim M J, Yeo J, Seo K I, Choi M S, Lee M K. Chlorogenic acid exhibits anti-obesity property and improves lipid metabolism in high-fat diet-induced-obese mice. Food Chem. Toxicol. 2010; 48:p.937–943.
80. Rivera L, Moron R, Sanchez M, Zarzuelo A, Galisteo M. Quercetin ameliorates metabolic syndrome and improves the inflammatory status in obese Zucker rats. *Obesity* (Silver Spring) 2008; 16:p.2081–2087.
81. Lim J, Iyer A, Liu L, Suen J Y, Lohman R J, Seow V, Yau M K, Brown L, Fairlie D P. Diet-induced obesity, adipose inflammation,

and metabolic dysfunction correlating with PAR2 expression are attenuated by PAR2 antagonism. *FASEB J.* 2013; December (27):p.4757-4767

82. Beltran-Sanchez, H et al "Prevalence and trends of metabolic syndrome in the adult US population, 1999-2010" *J Am Coll Cardiol.* 2013; Epub.
83. Ibid
84. Paliwal **R, Sharma V, Pracheta V. A review on Horse Radiah Tree (*Moringa oleifera*): A Multipurpose Tree with High Economic and Commercial Importance.** *Asian Journal of Biotechnology.* **2011;3(4):p.317-328.**
85. Thomsen M, Nordestgaard B G. "Myocardial Infarction and Ischemic Heart Disease in Overweight and Obesity With and Without Metabolic Syndrome." JAMA Intern Med. November 11, 2013.
86. Pan A, Sun Q, Bernstein A M, Manson J E, Willett W C, Hu F B. Changes in Red Meat Consumption and Subsequent Risk of Type 2 Diabetes MellitusThree Cohorts of US Men and Women. *JAMA Intern Med., 2013;* July 22(173(14):p.1328-1335.
87. Sutalangka C, Wattanathorn J, Muchimapura S, Thukhammee W. Moringa oleifera mitigates memory impairment and neurodegeneration in animal model of age-related dementia. Oxid Med Cell Longev. 2013;2013:695936
88. Hussain S, Malik F, Mahmood S.Review: An exposition of medicinal preponderance of *Moringa oleifera. Pak J Pharm Sci.* 2014 Mar;27(2):p.397-403.
89. Hannan M A, Kang J Y, Mohibbullah M, Hong Y K, Lee H, Choi J S, Choi I S, Moon I S. Moringa oleifera with promising neuronal survival and neurite outgrowth promoting potentials. J Ethnopharmacol. 2014 Feb 27;152(1):p142-150.
90. Chandra R K. Nutrition, immunity and infection: present knowledge and future directions. Lancet. 1983; 1: p.688-691.
91. WHO. Fifty-fifth World Health Assembly. Infant and Young Child Nutrition. Agenda Item 13.10. 18 May 2002.

92. Ruckmani K, Kavimani S, et al. Hepatoprotective activity of Moringa oleifera on antitubercular drug-induced liver damage in rats. Effect of Moringa oleifera Lam. on paracetamol-induced hepatotoxicity. Indian Journal of Pharmaceutical Sciences. 1998;60(1):p.33-35.
93. Rao K S, Misra S H. Anti-inflammatory and antihepatotoxic activities of the rats of Moringa pterygosperma. Geaertn Ind J Pharma Sci. 1998;60:p.12-16.
94. Paliwal R, Sharma V, Pracheta V, Sharma S H. Hepatoprotective and antioxidant potential of Moringa oleifera pods against DMBA-induced hepatocarcinogenesis in male mice. Int J Drug Dev Res. 2011c (in press).
95. NIH Record. NIH Celebrates Earth Day 2008. Vol LX. No.6. March 21, 2008. http://nihrecord.od.nih.gov/newsletters/2008/03_21_2008/story4.htm
96. Fahey J W. *Moringa oleifera*: a review of the medical evidence for its nutritional, therapeutic, and prophylactic properties. *Trees for Life Journal.* 2005;1(5) p. 1-13.
97. Paliwal **R, Sharma V, Pracheta V. A review on Horse Radiah Tree (*Moringa oleifera*): A Multipurpose Tree with High Economic and Commercial Importance. Asian Journal of Biotechnology. 2011;3(4):p.317-328.**
98. Fisher H W. *Moringa oleifera*: Magic, Myth or Miracle. Britannia Press. Toronto. 2011.
99. Kumar N A, Pari I. Antioxidant action of *Moringa oleifera* Lam (drumstick) against antitubercular drug induced lipid peroxidation in rats. *J Medicinal Foods.* 2003;6(3):p.255-259.
100. Bharali R, Tabassum J, Azad M R H. Chemomodulatory effect of *Moringa oleifera*, Lam, on hepatic carcinogen metabolizing enzymes, antioxidant parameters and skin papillomagenesis in mice. *Asian Pacific Journal of Cancer Prevention* 2003;4:p.131-139.
101. Njoku O U, Adikwu M U. Investigation on some physico-chemical antioxidant and toxicological properties of *Moringa oleifera* seed oil. *Acta Pharmaceutica Zagreb.* 1997;47(4): p.87-290.

102. Siddhuraju P, Becker K. Antioxidant properties of various solvent extracts of total phenolic constituents from three different agroclimatic origins of drumstick tree (*Moringa oleifera* Lam.) leaves. *Journal of Agricultural and Food Chemistry.* 2003;51:p.2144-2155.
103. National Pollution Prevention and Toxics Advisory Committee, Broader Issues Working Group, Initial thought starter: How can the EPA more efficiently identify potential risks and facilitate risk-reduction decisions for non-HPV chemicals? (October 6, 2005)
104. Philipson T J, Thornton Snider J, Lakdawalla D N, Stryckman B, Goldman D P. Impact of Oral Nutritional Supplementation on Hospital Outcomes. American Journal of Managed Care 2013;19(2):p.121-128.
105. Larsson, N. G. Somatic mitochondrial DNA mutations in mammalian aging. *Annu. Rev. Biochem.* 2010;**79**, p.683–706.
106. Ross J M., Stewart J B, Hagström E, Brene S, Mourier A, Freyer C, Lagouge M, Hoffer B J, Olson L Larsson N G. Germline mitochondrial DNA mutations aggravate ageing and can impair brain development. *Nature.* 2013; 21 August:p.412-415.
107. Chen Q, Vazquez E J, Moghaddas S, Hoppel C L, Lesnefsky E J. Production of reactive oxygen species by mitochondria: central role of complex III. *J Biol Chem.* 2003;Sep 19:278(38):p.36027-31
108. Njajou O T, Hsueh W C, Blackburn E H, et al. Association between telomere length, specific causes of death, and years of healthy life in health, aging, and body composition: a population-based cohort study. *J Gerontol A Biol Sci Med Sci.* 2009;64(8):p.860–864.
109. Cawthon R M, Smith K R, O'Brien E, Sivatchenko A, Kerber R A. Association between telomere length in blood and mortality in people aged 60 years or older. *Lancet.* 2003;361(9355):p.393–395.
110. Farzaneh-Far R, Lin J, Epel E S, Harris W S, Blackburn E H, Whooley M A. Association of Marine Omega-3 Fatty Acid Levels With Telomeric aging in Patients With Coronary Heart Disease. JAMA. Jan 20, 2010;303(3):p.250=257.

111. *Kiecolt-Glaser* J K, Epel E S, Belury M A, Andridge R, Lin J, Glaser R, Malarkey W B, Hwang B S, Blackburn E H. Omega-3 fatty acids, oxidative stress, and leukocyte telomere length: A randomized controlled trial. Brain Behav Immun. 2013; Feb;28:p.16-24
112. Aviv A. Telomeres and human somatic fitness. *J. Gerontol. Ser. A: Biol. Sci. Med. Sci.* 2006;61:p. 871–873.
113. Carrero J, Stenvinkel P, Fellstrom B, Qureshi A R, Lamb K, Heimburger O, Barany P, Radhakrishnan K, Lindholm B, Soveri I, Nordfors L, Shiels P G. Telomere attrition is associated with inflammation, low fetuin-a levels and high mortality in prevalent haemodialysis patients. *J. Intern Med.* 2008;263:p.302–312.
114. Damjanovic A K, Yang Y, Glaser R, Kiecolt-Glaser J K, Nguyen H, Laskowski B, Zou, Y, Beversdorf D Q, Weng N. Accelerated telomere erosion is associated with a declining immune function of caregivers of Alzheimer's disease patients. *J. Immunol.* 2007; 179:p.4249–4254.
115. Ornish D, Lin J, Chan J M, Epel E, Kemp C, Weidner G, Marlin R, Frenda S J, Magbanua M J M, Daubenmier J, Estay I, Hills N K, Chainani-Wu N, Carroll P R, Blackburn E H. Effect of comprehensive lifestyle changes on telomerase activity and telomere length in men with biopsy-proven low-risk prostate cancer: 5-year follow-up of a descriptive pilot study. Lancet. www.thelancet.com/oncology Published online September 17, 2013.
116. Stonehouse W, Conlon C A, Podd J, Hill S R, Minihane A M, Haskell C Kennedy D. Omega-3 Fatty Acids. University of Maryland Medical Center, Complementary and Alternative Medicine Guide. ISSFAL 2012.
117. **Kerti AV, Hermannstädter H M et al. Long-Chain Omega-3 Fatty Acids Improve Brain Function and Structure in Older Adults. *Cerebral Cortex*. Oxford University Journals, June 24, 2013.**
118. Nikolakopoulou Z, Nteliopoulos G, Michael-Titus A T, Parkinson E K. Omega-3 polyunsaturated fatty acids selectively inhibit growth in neoplastic oral keratinocytes by differentially activating ERK1/2." *Carcinogenesis*; 2013; 34 (12): p.2716-2725.

119. Moyo B, Masika P J, Hugo A, Muchenje V. Nutritional characterization of Moringa (*Moringa oleifera* **Lam.**) leaves. African Journal of Biotechnology. 2011; October 5. Vol.10 (60), p. 12925-12933.
120. Sanchez-Machado DI, Nunez-Gastelum JA, Reyes-Moreno C, Ramirez-Wong B, Lopenz-Cervantes J. Nutritional Quality of edible Parts of *Moringa oleifera*. *Food Anal Method.* 2009; DOI 10.1007/s1261-009-9106-Z.
121. Solivaa C R, Kreuzera M, Foidlb N, Foidlb G, A. Machmuller A. Feeding value of whole and extracted *Moringa oleifera* leaves for ruminants and their effects on ruminal fermentation in vitro. *Animal Feed Science and Technology.* 2005;p.118 47–62
122. Aben A, Danckaerts M. Omega-3 and omega-6 fatty acids in the treatment of children and adolescents with ADHD. *Tijdschr Psychiatr.* 2010; 52(2):p.89-97.
123. Buckley M S, Goff A D, Knapp W E, et al. Fish oil interaction with warfarin. *Ann Pharmacother.* 2004;38:50-2.
124. Burgess J, Stevens L, Zhang W, Peck L. Long-chain polyunsaturated fatty acids in children with attention-deficit hyperactivity disorder. *Am J Clin Nutr.* 2000; 71(suppl):p.327S-330S.
125. Dopheide J A, Pliszka S R. Attention-deficit-hyperactivity disorder: an update. *Pharmacotherapy.* 2009 Jun;29(6):p.656-79.
126. Mattar M, Obeid O. Fish oil and the management of hypertriglyceridemia. *Nutr Health.* 2009;20(1):41-9.
127. Mitchell EA, Aman MG, Turbott SH, Manku M. Clinical characteristics and serum essential fatty acid levels in hyperactive children. *Clin Pediatr* (Phila). 1987;26:p.406-411.
128. Richardson A J, Puri B K. The potential role of fatty acids in attention-deficit/hyperactivity disorder. *Prostaglandins Leukot Essent Fatty Acids.* 2000;63(1/2):p.79-87.
129. Nagakura T, Matsuda S, Shichijyo K, Sugimoto H, Hata K. Dietary supplementation with fish oil rich in omega-3 polyunsaturated fatty acids in children with bronchial asthma. *Eur Resp J.* 2000;16(5):p.861-865.

130. Okamoto M, Misunobu F, Ashida K, et al. Effects of dietary supplementation with n-3 fatty acids compared with n-6 fatty acids on bronchial asthma. *Int Med.* 2000;39(2):p.107-111.
131. Cole G M. Omega-3 fatty acids and dementia. *Prostaglandins Leukot Essent Fatty Acids.* 2009; 81(2-3):p.213-21.
132. Complementary and Alternative Medicine for the Treatment of Depressive Disorders in Women. *Psychiatric Clinics of North America.* 2010;p.33(2).
133. Frangou S, Lewis M, McCrone P et al. Efficacy of ethyl-eicosapentaenoic acid in bipolar depression: randomised double-blind placebo-controlled study. *Br J Psychiatry.* 2006;p.188:p.46-50
134. Rocha Araujo D M, Vilarim M M, Nardi A E. What is the effectiveness of the use of polyunsaturated fatty acid omega-3 in the treatment of depression? *Expert Rev Neurother.* 2010; 10(7):p.1117-29.
135. Sarris J, Schoendorfer N, Kavanagh DJ. Major depressive disorder and nutritional medicine: a review of monotherapies and adjuvant treatments. *Nutr Rev.* 2009 Mar;67(3):p.125-31. Review.
136. Silvers K M, Woolley C C, Hamilton F C et al. Randomised double-blind placebo-controlled trial of fish oil in the treatment of depression. *Prostaglandins Leukot Essent Fatty Acids.* 2005;72:p.211-8.
137. Stark KD, Park EJ, Maines VA, et al. Effect of fish-oil concentrate on serum lipids in postmenopausal women receiving and not receiving hormone replacement therapy in a placebo-controlled, double blind trial. *Am J Clin Nutr.* 2000;72:p.389-394.
138. Aronson W J, Glaspy J A, Reddy S T, Reese D, Heber D, Bagga D. Modulation of omega-3/omega-6 polyunsaturated ratios with dietary fish oils in men with prostate cancer. *Urology.* 2001;58(2):p.283-288.
139. Daniel C R, McCullough M L, Patel R C, Jacobs E J, Flanders W D, Thun M J, Calle E E. Dietary intake of omega-6 and omega-3 fatty acids and risk of colorectal cancer in a prospective cohort of U.S. men and women. *Cancer Epidemiol Biomarkers Prev.* 2009 Feb;18(2):p.516-25.

140. Freeman V L, Meydani M, Yong S, Pyle J, Flanigan R C, Waters W B, Wojcik E M. Prostatic levels of fatty acids and the histopathology of localized prostate cancer. *J Urol.* 2000;164(6):p.2168-2172.
141. Hall M N, Campos H, Li H, Sesso H D, Stampfer M J, Willett W C, Ma J. Blood levels of long-chain polyunsaturated fatty acids, aspirin, and the risk of colorectal cancer. *Cancer Epidemiol Biomarkers Prev.* 2007;16(2):p.314-21.
142. Newcomer L M, King I B, Wicklund K G, Stanford J L. The association of fatty acids with prostate cancer risk. *Prostate.* 2001;47(4):p.262-268.
143. Nikolakopoulou Z, Nteliopoulos G, Michael-Titus A T, Parkinson E K. Omega-3 polyunsaturated fatty acids selectively inhibit growth in neoplastic oral keratinocytes by differentially activating ERK1/2." Carcinogenesis; 2013; 34 (12): 2716-2725.
144. LichtensteinT P, Feychting M, Ahlbom A, Wolk A. Fatty fish consumption and risk of prostate cancer. *Lancet.* 2001; 357(9270) :p.1764-1766.
145. Fotuhi M, Mohassel P, Yaffe K. Fish consumption, long-chain omega-3 fatty acids and risk of cognitive decline or Alzheimer disease: a complex association. *Nat Clin Pract Neurol.* 2009 Mar;5(3):p.140-52. Review.
146. Freund-Levi Y F, Eriksdotter-Jonhagen M, Cederholm T, et al. Omega-3 fatty acid treatment in 174 patients with mild to moderate Alzheimer disease: OmegAD Study. *Arch Neurol.* 2006;63:p.1402-8.
147. Freund-Levi Y, Hjorth E, Lindberg C, Cederholm T, Faxen-Irving G, Vedin I, Palmblad J, Wahlund LO, Schultzberg M, Basun H, Eriksdotter Jönhagen M. Effects of omega-3 fatty acids on inflammatory markers in cerebrospinal fluid and plasma in Alzheimer's disease: the OmegAD study. *Dement Geriatr Cogn Disord.* 2009;27(5):p.481-90.
148. **Witte A V, Kerti L, Hermannstädter H M et al. "Long-Chain Omega-3 Fatty Acids Improve Brain Function and Structure in Older Adults." Cerebral Cortex, Oxford University Journals, June 24, 2013.**

149. Montori V, Farmer A, Wollan PC, Dinneen SF. Fish oil supplementation in type 2 diabetes: a quantitative systematic review. *Diabetes Care.* 2000;23:p.1407-1415.
150. Angerer P, von Schacky C. n-3 polyunsaturated fatty acids and the cardiovascular system. *Curr Opin Lipidol.* 2000;11(1):p.57-63.
151. Balk EM, Lichtenstein AH, Chung M et al. Effects of omega-3 fatty acids on serum markers of cardiovascular disease risk: A systematic review. *Atherosclerosis.* 2006 Nov;189(1):p.19-30.
152. Calo L, Bianconi L, Colivicchi F et al. N-3 Fatty acids for the prevention of atrial fibrillation after coronary artery bypass surgery: a randomized, controlled trial. *J Am Coll Cardiol.* 2005;45:p.1723-8.
153. Caron MF, White CM. Evaluation of the antihyperlipidemic properties of dietary supplements. *Pharmacotherapy.* 2001;21(4):p.481-487.
154. Chattipakorn N, Settakorn J, Petsophonsakul P, et al. Cardiac mortality is associated with low levels of omega-3 and omega-6 fatty acids in the heart of cadavers with a history of coronary heart disease.*Nutr Res.* 2009; 29(10);p.696-704.
155. Christensen JH, Skou HA, Fog L, Hansen V, Vesterlund T, Dyerberg J, Toft E, Schmidt EB. Marine n-3 fatty acids, wine intake, and heart rate variability in patients referred for coronary angiography. *Circulation.* 2001;103:p.623-625.
156. Dewailly E, Blanchet C, Lemieux S, et al. n-3 fatty acids and cardiovascular disease risk factors among the Inuit of Nunavik. *Am J Clin Nutr.* 2001;74(4):p.464-473.
157. Fatty fish consumption and ischemic heart disease mortality in older adults: The cardiovascular heart study. Presented at the American Heart Association's 41st annual conference on cardiovascular disease epidemiology and prevention. AHA. 2001.
158. Galli C, Risé P. Fish consumption, omega 3 fatty acids and cardiovascular disease. The science and the clinical trials. *Nutr Health.* 2009;20(1):p.11-20. Review.
159. Geelen A, Brouwer IA, Schouten EG et al. Effects of n-3 fatty acids from fish on premature ventricular complexes and heart rate in humans. *Am J Clin Nutr.* 2005;81:p.416-20.

160. Hooper L, Thompson R, Harrison R et al. Omega 3 fatty acids for prevention and treatment of cardiovascular disease. *Cochrane Database Syst Rev.* 2004;CD003177.
161. Iso H, Rexrode K M, Stampfer M J, Manson J E, Colditz G A, Speizer F E et al. Intake of fish and omega-3 fatty acids and risk of stroke in women. *JAMA.* 2001;285(3):p.304-312.
162. Hartweg J, Farmer AJ, Holman RR, Neil A. Potential impact of omega-3 treatment on cardiovascular disease in type 2 diabetes. *Curr Opin Lipidol.* 2009 Feb;20(1):p.30-8.
163. Kelley DS, Siegel D, Fedor DM, Adkins Y, Mackey BE. DHA supplementation decreases serum C-reactive protein and other markers of inflammation in hypertriglyceridemic men. *J Nutr.* 2009 Mar;139(3):p.495-501.
164. Krauss R M, Eckel R H, Howard B, et al. AHA Scientific Statement: AHA Dietary guidelines Revision 2000: A statement for healthcare professionals from the nutrition committee of the American Heart Association. *Circulation.* 2000;102(18):p.2284-2299.
165. Kris-Etherton P, Eckel R H, Howard B V, St. Jeor S, Bazzare TL. AHA Science Advisory: Lyon Diet Heart Study. Benefits of a Mediterranean-style, National Cholesterol Education Program/American Heart Association Step I Dietary Pattern on Cardiovascular Disease. *Circulation.* 2001; p.103:1823.
166. Lee J H, O'Keefe J H, Lavie C J; Harris W S. Omega-3 fatty acids: cardiovascular benefits, sources and sustainability. *Nat Rev Cardiol.* 2009; 6(12):p.753-8.
167. Mori T A. Omega-3 fatty acids and blood pressure. *Cell Mol Biol (Nosiy-le-grand).* 2010; 56(1):p.83-92.
168. Mozaffarian D, Geelen A, Brouwer I A et al. Effect of Fish Oil on Heart Rate in Humans. A Meta-Analysis of Randomized Controlled Trials. *Circulation.* 2005;112(13):p.1945-52.
169. Miller P E, Van Elswyk M V, Alexander D D. Long-Chain Omega-3 Fatty Acids Eicosapentaenoic Acid and Docosahexaenoic Acid and Blood Pressure: A Meta-Analysis of Randomized Controlled Trials. Am J Hypertens. March 6, 2014.

170. Belluzzi A, Boschi S, Brignola C, Munarini A, Cariani C, Miglio F. Polyunsaturated fatty acids and inflammatory bowel disease. *Am J Clin Nutr.* 2000;71(suppl):p.339S-342S.
171. Dichi I, Frenhane P, Dichi J B, Correa C R, Angeleli A Y, Bicudo M H, et al. Comparison of omega-3 fatty acids and sulfasalazine in ulcerative colitis. *Nutrition.* 2000;16:p.87-90.
172. Geerling BJ, Badart-Smook A, van Deursen C, et al. Nutritional supplementation with N-3 fatty acids and antioxidants in patients with Crohn's disease in remission: effects on antioxidant status and fatty acid profile. *Inflamm Bowel Dis.* 2000;6(2):p.77-84.
173. Romano C, Cucchiara S, Barabino A et al. Usefulness of omega-3 fatty acid supplementation in addition to mesalazine in maintaining remission in pediatric Crohn's disease: A double-blind, randomized, placebo-controlled study. *World J Gastroenterol.* 2006; 11: p.7118-21.
174. Cho E, Hung S, Willet W C, Spiegelman D, Rimm E B, Seddon J M, et al. Prospective study of dietary fat and the risk of age-related macular degeneration. *Am J Clin Nutr.* 2001;73(2):p.209-218.
175. Seddon J M, Rosner B, Sperduto R D, Yannuzzi L, Haller J A, Blair N P, Willett W. Dietary fat and risk for advanced age-related macular degeneration. *Arch Opthalmol.* 2001;119(8):p.1191-1199.
176. Smith W, Mitchell P, Leeder S R. Dietary fat and fish intake and age-related maculopathy. *Arch Opthamol.* 2000; 118(3): p.401-404.
177. Fenton WS, Dicerson F, Boronow J, et al. A placebo controlled trial of omega-3 fatty acid (ethyl eicosapentaenoic acid) supplementation for residual symptoms and cognitive impairment in schizophrenia. *Am J Psychiatry.* 2001;158(12):p.2071-2074.
178. Joy C B, Mumby-Croft R, Joy L A. Polyunsaturated fatty acid supplementation for schizophrenia. *Cochrane Database Syst Rev.* 2006 Jul 19;3:CD001257. Review.
179. Bahadori B, Uitz E, Thonhofer R, et al. omega-3 Fatty acids infusions as adjuvant therapy in rheumatoid arthritis. *JPEN J Parenter Enteral Nutr.* 2010; 34(2):p.151-5.

180. Berbert AA, Kondo CR, Almendra CL et al. Supplementation of fish oil and olive oil in patients with rheumatoid arthritis. *Nutrition.* 2005;21:p.131-6.
181. Di Giuseppe D, Wallin A, Bottai M, Askling J, Wolk A. Long-term intake of dietary long-chain n-3 polyunsaturated fatty acids and risk of rheumatoid arthritis: a prospective cohort study of women. *Ann Rheum Dis 2013*
182. Hagen KB, Byfuglien MG, Falzon L, Olsen SU, Smedslund G. Dietary interventions for rheumatoid arthritis. *Cochrane Database Syst Rev.* 2009 Jan 21;(1):CD006400. Review.
183. Kremer JM. N-3 fatty acid supplements in rheumatoid arthritis. *Am J Clin Nutr.* 2000;(suppl 1):p.349S-351S.
184. Boelsma E, Hendriks HF. Roza L. Nutritional skin care: health effects of micronutrients and fatty acids. *Am J Clin Nutr.* 2001;73(5):p.853-864.
185. Bradbury J, Myers S P, Oliver C et al. An adaptogenic role for omega-3 fatty acids in stress; a randomised placebo controlled double blind intervention study (pilot)ISRCTN22569553. *Nutr J.* 2004 Nov 28;3:p.20.
186. Berson E L, Rosner B, Sandberg M A, et al. Clinical trial of docosahexaenoic acid in patients with retinitis pigmentosa receiving vitamin A treatment. *Arch Ophthalmol.* 2004;122(9):p.1297-1305.
187. Chan EJ, Cho L. What can we expect from omega-3 fatty acids? *Cleve Clin J Med.* 2009 Apr;76(4):245-51. Review.
188. Goldberg R J, Katz J. A meta-analysis of the analgesic effects of omega-3 polyunsaturated fatty acid supplementation for inflammatory joint pain. *Pain.* 2007 Feb 28
189. Itomura M, Hamazaki K, Sawazaki S et al. The effect of fish oil on physical aggression in schoolchildren - a randomized, double-blind, placebo-controlled trial. *J Nutr Biochem.* 2005;16:p.163-71.
190. Jeschke M G, Herndon D N, Ebener C, Barrow R E, Jauch K W. Nutritional intervention high in vitamins, protein, amino acids, and omega-3 fatty acids improves protein metabolism

during the hypermetabolic state after thermal injury. *Arch Surg.* 2001;136:p.1301-1306.
191. Olsen SF, Secher NJ. Low consumption of seafood in early pregnancy as a risk factor for preterm delivery: prospective cohort study. *BMJ.* 2002;324(7335):p. 447-451.
192. Riediger N D, Othman R A, Suh M, Moghadasian M H. A systemic review of the roles of n-3 fatty acids in health and disease. *J Am Diet Assoc.* 2009 Apr;109(4):p.668-79. Review.
193. Sundstrom B, Stalnacke K, Hagfors L et al. Supplementation of omega-3 fatty acids in patients with ankylosing spondylitis. *Scand J Rheumatol.* 2006;35:p.359-62.
194. Weinstock-Guttman B, Baier M, Park Y et al. Low fat dietary intervention with omega-3 fatty acid supplementation in multiple sclerosis patients. *Prostaglandins Leukot Essent Fatty Acids.* 2005;73:p.397-404.
195. Yashodhara BM. Omega-3 fatty acids: a comprehensive review of their role in health and disease. *Postgrad Med J.* 2009; 85(1000):p.84-90.
196. Yuen AW, Sander JW, Fluegel D et al. Omega-3 fatty acid supplementation in patients with chronic epilepsy: A randomized trial. *Epilepsy Behav.* 2005;7(2):p.253-8.
197. Tousoulis D, Plastiras A, Siasos G, Oikonomou E, Verveniotis A, Kokkou E, Maniatis K, Gouliopoulos N, Miliou A, Paraskevopoulos T, Stefanadis C. Omega-3 PUFAs improved endothelial function and arterial stiffness with a parallel antiinflammatory effect in adults with metabolic syndrome. Atherosclerosis. 2014 Jan; 232(1) :p.10-6.
198. American College of Sports Medicine: American College of Sports Medicine position stand. Progression models in resistance training for healthy adults. *Med Sci Sports Exerc.* 2009;41:p.687-708.
199. Kraemer W J, Ratamess N A. Fundamentals of resistance training: progression and exercise prescription. *Med Sci Sports Exerc.* 2004; 36:p.674-688.

200. Ha E, Zemel M B. Functional properties of whey, whey components, and essential amino acids: mechanisms underlying health benefits for active people (review). *J Nutr Biochem.* 2003; 14:p.251-258.
201. Tipton K D, Rasmussen B B, Miller S L, Wolf S E, Owens-Stovall S K, Petrini B E, Wolfe R R. Timing of amino acid-carbohydrate ingestion alters anabolic response of muscle to resistance exercise. *Am J Physiol Endocrinol Metab* 2001; 281:p.E197-206.
202. Beelen M, Burke L M, Gibala M J, van Loon L J C. Nutritional strategies to promote postexercise recovery. *Int J Sport Exerc Metab.* 2010; December 20(6):p.515-532.
203. Howarth K R, Moreau N A, Phillips S M, Gibala M J. Coingestion of protein with carbohydrate during recovery from endurance exercise stimulates skeletal muscle protein synthesis in humans. *J Appl Phsiol.* 2009; April 106(4):p.1394-1402.
204. Kerksick C M, Rasmussen C J, Lancaster S L, Magu B, Smith P, Melton C, Greenwood M, Almada A L, Earnest C P, Kreider R B: The effects of protein and amino acid supplementation on performance and training adaptations during ten weeks of resistance training. *J Strength Cond Res* 2006, 20:p.643-653.
205. Häussinger D. The role of cellular hydration in the regulation of cell function. *Biochem J.* 1996; 313:p.607-710.
206. Kimball S R. The role of nutrition in stimulating muscle protein accretion at the molecular level. *Biochem Soc Trans* 2007; 35:p.1298-1301.
207. Batmanghelidj F. Your Body's Many Cries for Water: A Preventive and Self-Education Manual for Those Who Prefer to Adhere to the Logic of the Natural and the Simple in Medicine. Global Health Solutions. Falls Church, VA. 1995.
208. Willoughby D S, Stout J R, Wilborn C D. Effects of resistance training and protein plus amino acid supplementation on muscle anabolism, mass, and strength. *Amino Acids.*2007; 32:p.467-477.
209. Volek J. Influence of nutrition on responses to resistance training. *Med Sci Sports Exerc.* 2004;36:p.689-696.

210. Anwar F, Latif S, Ashraf M, Gilani A H, *Moringa oleifera*: a food plant with multiple medicinal uses. *Phytother Res.* 2007; 21(1): p.17-25.
211. Fahey J W. *Moringa oleifera*: a review of the medical evidence for its nutritional, therapeutic, and prophylactic properties. *Trees for Life Journal.* 2005;1(5) p. 1-13.
212. Paliwal **R, Sharma V, Pracheta V. A review on Horse Radiah Tree (Moringa oleifera): A Multipurpose Tree with High Economic and Commercial Importance. Asian Journal of Biotechnology. 2011;3(4):p.317-328.**
213. Fisher H W. *Moringa* Oleifera: Magic, Myth or Miracle. Britannia Press. Toronto. 2011.
214. Biolo G, Tipton KD, Klein S, Wolfe RR: An abundant supply of amino acids enhances the metabolic effect of exercise on muscle protein. *Am J Physiol* 1997, 273:p.E122-9.
215. Biolo G, Maggi S P, Williams B D, Tipton K D, Wolfe R R. Increased rates of muscle protein turnover and amino acid transport after resistance exercise in humans. *Am J Physiol.* 1995;268:p.E514-520.
216. Tipton K D, Wolfe R R. Exercise, protein metabolism and muscle growth. *Int J Sport Nutr Exerc Metab.* 2001;Mar:11(1):p.109-132.
217. Andersen L L, Tufekovic G, Zebis M K, Crameri R M, Verlaan G, Kjaer M, Suetta C, Magnusson P, Aagaard P. The effect of resistance training combined with timed ingestion of protein on muscle fiber size and muscle strength. *Metabolism.* 2005;54(2):p.151-156.
218. Phillips S M, Hartman J W, Wilkinson S B. Dietary protein to support anabolism with resistance exercise in young men. *J Am Coll Nutr.* 2005; Apr 24(2):p.134S-139S.
219. Levenhagen DK, Gresham JD, Carlson MG, Maron DJ, Borel MJ, Flakoll PJ: Postexercise nutrient intake timing in humans is critical to recovery of leg glucose and protein homeostasis. *Am J Physiol Endocrinol Metab* 2001, 280:p.E982-93.
220. Tipton K D, Rasmussen B B, Miller S L, Wolf S E, Owens-Stovall S K, Petrini B E, Wolfe R R. Timing of amino acid-carbohydrate ingestion alters anabolic response of muscle to resistance exercise. *Am J Physiol Endocrinol Metab* 2001; 281:p.E197-206.

221. Kerksick C, Harvey T, Stout J, Campbell B, Wilborn C, Kreider R, Kalman D, Ziegenfuss T, Lopez H, Landis J, Ivy JL, Antonio J: International Society of Sports Nutrition position stand: Nutrient timing. *J Int Soc Sports Nutr* 2008;5:p.17.
222. Cribb P J, Hayes A. Effects of supplement timing and resistance exercise on skeletal muscle hypertrophy. *Med Sci Sports Exerc.* 2006; 38:p.1918-1925.
223. Volek J S. General nutritional considerations for strength athletes. Nutrition and the Strength Athlete, C. Jackson (Ed). Boca Raton, FL. CRC Press. 2000.
224. Hoffman JR, Ratamess NA, Tranchina CP, Rashti SL, Kang J, Faigenbaum AD: Effect of a proprietary protein supplement on recovery indices following resistance exercise in strength/power athletes. *Amino Acids.* 2010; 38:p.771-778
225. Hoffman J R, Ratamess N A, Tranchina C P, Rashti S L, Kang J, Faigenbaum A D. Effect of a proprietary protein supplement on recovery indices following resistance exercise in strength/power athletes. *Amino Acids* 2010, 38:p.771-778.
226. Roy B D, Tarnopolsky M A, MacDougal J D, Fowles J, Yarasheski K E. effect of glucose supplement timing on protein metabolism after resistance training. *J Appl Physiol.* 1997;82:p.1882-1888.
227. Moore D R, Tang J E, Burd N A, Rerecich T, Tarnopolsky M A, Phillips S M. Differential stimulation of myofibrillar and sarcoplasmic protein synthesis with protein ingestion at rest and after resistance exercise. *J Physiol.* 2009;587:p.897-904.
228. Drummond M J, Dreyer H C, Fry C S, Glynn E L, Rasmussen B B. Nutritional and contractile regulation of human skeletal muscle protein synthesis and mTORC1 signaling. *J Appl Physiol.* 2009;Apr 106(4):p.1374-1384.
229. Moore D R, Tang J E, Burd N A, Rerecich T, Tarnopolsky M A, Phillips S M. Differential stimulation of myofibrillar and sarcoplasmic protein synthesis with protein ingestion at rest and after resistance exercise. *J Physiol.* 2009;587:p.897-904.

230. Kraemer W J, Adams K, Cafarelli E, Dudley G A, Dooly C, Feigenbaum M S, Fleck S J, Franklin B, Fry A C, Hoffman J R, Newton R U, Potteiger J, Stone M H, Ratamess N A, Triplett-McBride T. American College of **Sports Medicine position stand. Progression models in resistance training for healthy adults.** *Med Sci Sports Exerc.* 2002;34:p.364-380.

231. Hullmi J J, Ahtiainen J P, Kaasalainen T, Pöllänen E, Häkkinen K, Alen M, Selänne H, Kovanen V, Mero AA. Postexercise myostatin and activin IIb mRNA levels: effects of strength training. *Med Sci Sports Exerc* 2007;39:p.289-297.

232. Kraemer W J, Ratamess N A. **Fundamentals of resistance training: progression and exercise prescription.** *Med Sci Sports Exerc.* 2004;36:p.674-688.

233. Hulmi J J, Kovenen V, Selänne H, Kraemer W J, Häkkinen K, Mero A A. Acute and long-term effects of resistance exercise with or without protein ingestion on muscle hypertrophy and gene expression. *Amino Acids.* 2009;37:p.297-308.

234. Volek J. Influence of nutrition on responses to resistance training. *Med Sci Sports Exerc.* 2004;36:p.689-696.

235. Kerksick C, Harvey T, Stout J, Campbell B, Wilborn C, Kreider R, Kalman D, Ziegenfuss T, Lopez H, Landis J, Ivy JL, Antonio J: International Society of Sports Nutrition position stand: Nutrient timing. *J Int Soc Sports Nutr* 2008;5:p.17.

236. Bird S P, Tarpenning K M, Marino F E. Liquid carbohydrate/essential amino acid ingestion during a short-term bout of resistance exercise suppresses myofibrillar protein degradation. *Metabolism* 2006;55:p.570-577.

237. Bennet W M, Conacher A A, Scrimgeor C M, Smith K, Bennie M J. Increase in anterior tibialis muscle protein synthesis in healthy man during mixed amino acid infusion: studies of incorporation of [1- 13C] leucine. *Clin Sci (Colch).* 1989; 76:p.447-454.

238. Rasmussen B B, Tipton K D, Miller S L, Wolf S E, Wolfe R R. An oral amino acid-carbohydrate supplement enhances muscle protein

anabolism after resistance training overreaching. *J Strength Cond Res.* 2003;17:p.250-258.
239. Biolo G, Tipton KD, Klein S, Wolfe RR: An abundant supply of amino acids enhances the metabolic effect of exercise on muscle protein. *Am J Physiol* 1997, 273:p.E122-9.
240. Abdulkarim S M, Long K, Lai O M, Muhammad S K S, Ghalazi H M. Some physic-chemical properties of *Moringa oleifera* seed oil extracted using solvent and aqueous enzymatic methods. *Food Chem.* 2005;93:p.253-263.
241. Makkar H P S, Becker K. Nutrients and antiquality factors in different morphological parts of the *Moringa oleifera* tree. *Journal of Agricultural Science, Cambridge* (1997);128:p. 31-322.
242. Kraemer W J, Ratamess N A, Volek J S, Häkkinen K, Rubin M R, French D N, Gómez A L, McGuigan M R, Scheett T P, Newton R U, Spiering B A, Izquierdo M, Dioguardi F S. The effects of amino acid supplementation on hormonal response to resistance training overreaching. *Metabolism.* 2006; Mar 55(3):p.282-291
243. Volek J. Influence of nutrition on responses to resistance training. *Med Sci Sports Exerc.* 2004;36:p.689-696.
244. Biolo G, Tipton KD, Klein S, Wolfe RR: An abundant supply of amino acids enhances the metabolic effect of exercise on muscle protein. *Am J Physiol* 1997, 273:p.E122-9.
245. Hulmi J J, Kovanen V, Selänne H, Kraemer WJ, Häkkinen K, Mero A A. Acute and long-term effects of resistance exercise with or without protein ingestion on muscle hypertrophy and gene expression. *Amino Acids* 2009, 37:p.297-308.
246. Haub M D, Wells A M, Tarnopolsky M A, Campbell W W. Effect of protein source on resistive-training-induced changes in body composition and muscle size in older men. *Am J Clin Nutr* 2002;76:p.511-517.
247. Tipton K D, Rasmussen B B, Miller S L, Wolf S E, Owens-Stovall S K, Petrini B E, Wolfe R R. Timing of amino acid-carbohydrate ingestion alters anabolic response of muscle to resistance exercise. *Am J Physiol Endocrinol Metab* 2001, 281:p.E197-206.

248. Esmarck B, Andersen J L, Olsen S, Richter E A, Mizuno M, Kjaer M: Timing of postexercise protein intake is important for muscle hypertrophy with resistance training in elderly humans. *J Physiol* 2001; 535:p.301-311.
249. Borsheim E, Tipton K D, Wolf S E, Wolfe R R. Essential amino acids and muscle protein recovery from resistance exercise. *Am J Physiol Endocrinol Metab* 2002; 283:p.E648-57.
250. Cockburn E, Hayes P R, French D N, Stevenson E, St Clair Gibson A. Acute milk-based protein-CHO supplementation attenuates exercise-induced muscle damage. *Appl Physiol Nutr Metab* 2008; 33:p.775-783.
251. Naidoo K K, Coopoosamy R M. Review on herbal remedies used by the 1860 South African Indian settlers. *African J Biotech.* 2011;10 August:p.8533-8535.
252. Fahey J W. *Moringa oleifera*: a review of the medical evidence for its nutritional, therapeutic, and prophylactic properties. *Trees for Life Journal.* 2005;1(5) p. 1-13.
253. Fuglie L J. Combating Malnutrition with Moringa. Development Potential for Moringa Products. *Church World Service.* Oct 29 to Nov 2, 2001.
254. Makkar H P S, Becker K. Nutrients and antiquality factors in different morphological parts of the *Moringa oleifera* tree. *Journal of Agricultural Science, Cambridge* (1997);128:p. 31-322.
255. Johnson B C. Clinical Perspectives on the Health Effects of *Moringa* oleifera: A Promising Adjunct for Balanced Nutrition and Better Health. *KOS Health Publications.* 2005;Aug:p.1-5.
256. Sánchez-Machado D I, Núñez-Gastélum J A, Cuauhtémoc R M, Benjamin Ramírez-Wong B, López-Cervantes J. Nutritional Quality of Edible Parts of *Moringa* oleifera. *Food Analytical Methods.* 2010;3(3):p.175-180.
257. Hunter I R, Stewart J L. Foliar nutrient and nutritive content of central American multipurpose tree species growing at Comayagua, Honduras. *Commonwealth Forestry Review.* 1993; 72(3): p. 193-197.

258. Fahey J W. *Moringa oleifera*: a review of the medical evidence for its nutritional, therapeutic, and prophylactic properties. *Trees for Life Journal.* 2005;1(5) p. 1-13.
259. Martin F W, Ruberte R M, Meitzner L S. *Edible Leaves of the Tropics.* 3rd Ed. Educational Concerns for Hunger Organization Inc. N. Ft. Meyers, FL. 1998;194pp.
260. Borsheim E, Tipton K D, Wolf S E, Wolfe R R. Essential amino acids and muscle protein recovery from resistance exercise. *Am J Physiol Endocrinol Metab* 2002; 283:p.E648-57.
261. Moore D R, Robinson M J, Fry J L, Tang J E, Glover E I, Wilkinson S B, Prior T, Tarnopolsky M A, Phillips SM. Ingested protein dose response of muscle and albumin protein synthesis after resistance exercise in young men. *Am J Clin Nutr.* 2009,;89:p.161-168.
262. Volek J. Influence of nutrition on responses to resistance training. *Med Sci Sports Exerc.* 2004;36:p.689-696.
263. Symons T B, Sheffield-Moore M, Wolfe R R, Paddon-Jones D. A moderate serving of high-quality protein maximally stimulates skeletal muscle protein synthesis in young and elderly subjects. *J Am Diet Assoc.* 2009;109:p.1582-1586.
264. Ramachandran C, Peter K V, Gopalakrishnan P K. 1980, Drumstick (*Moringa* oleifera): A multipurpose Indian Vegetable. *Economic Botany,* 34 (3) p.276-283.
265. Bird S P, Tarpenning K M, Marino F E. Independent and combined effects of liquid carbohydrate/essential amino acid ingestion on hormonal and muscular adaptations following resistance training in untrained men. *Eur J Appl Physiol.* 2006;97:p.225-238.
266. Coyle E F, Coggan A R, Hemmert M K, Ivy J L. Muscle glycogen utilization during prolonged strenuous exercise when fed carbohydrate. *J Appl Physiol.* 1986;61:p.165-172.
267. Pascoe D D, Costill D L, Fink W J, Roberg R A, Zachweija J J. Glycogen resynthesis in skeletal muscle following resistive exercise. *Med Sci Sports Exerc.* 1993; 25:p.359-354.
268. Robergs R A, Pearson D R, Costill D L, Fink W J, Pascoe D D, Benedict M A, Lambert C P, Zachweija J J. Muscle glycogenolysis

during differing intensities of weight-resistance exercise. *J Appl Physiol.* 1991;70:p.1700-1706.
269. Hargreaves M, Costill D L, Coggan A R, Fink W J, Nishibata I. Effect of carbohydrate feedings on muscle glycogen utilization and exercise performance. Med Sci Sports Exerc. 1984;16:p.219-222
270. Coggan A R, Coyle E F. Carbohydrate ingestion during prolonged exercise: effects on metabolism and performance. *Exerc Sport Sci Rev.* 1991;19:p.1-40.
271. Haff G G, Lehmkuhl M J, McCoy L B, Stone M H. Carbohydrate supplementation and resistance training. *J StrengthCond Res.* 2003; Feb 17(1):p.187-196.
272. Kerksick C, Harvey T, Stout J, Campbell B, Wilborn C, Kreider R, Kalman D, Ziegenfuss T, Lopez H, Landis J, Ivy JL, Antonio J: International Society of Sports Nutrition position stand: Nutrient timing. *J Int Soc Sports Nutr* 2008;5:p.17.
273. Hargreaves M, Costill D L, Coggan A R, Fink W J, Nishibata I. Effect of carbohydrate feedings on muscle glycogen utilization and exercise performance. Med Sci Sports Exerc. 1984;16:p.219-222
274. ibid
275. Coggan AR, Coyle EF (1991) Carbohydrate ingestion during prolonged exercise: effects on metabolism and performance. Exerc Sport Sci Rev 19:p.1-40
276. Conley M S, Stone M H. Carbohydrate ingestion/supplementation or resistance exercise and training 1996;21(1):p. 7-17
277. Ratamess N A, Kraemer W J, Volek J V, Harman M J S, McGuigan M M, Scheett T. The effects of amino acid supplementation on muscular performance during resistance training. *J Strength & Cond Res.* (2003;17(2):p.250-258.
278. Robergs R A. Nutrition and exercise determinants of postexercise glycogen synthesis. *Int J Sport Nutr.* 1991;Dec 1 (4):p.307-337.
279. Coyle E F, Coggan A R, Hemmert M K, Ivy J L. Muscle glycogen utilization during prolonged strenuous exercise when fed carbohydrate. *J Appl Physiol.* 1986; Jul;61(1):p.165-72.

280. Kerksick C, Harvey T, Stout J, Campbell B, Wilborn C, Kreider R, Kalman D, Ziegenfuss T, Lopez H, Landis J, Ivy JL, Antonio J: International Society of Sports Nutrition position stand: Nutrient timing. *J Int Soc Sports Nutr* 2008;5:p.17.
281. Nazar K, Brzezinska Z, Kowalski W. Mechanism of impaired capacity for muscular work following Beta-adrenergic blockade in dogs. *Pfuegers Arch.* 1972;336:p.72-78.
282. Mustapha P, Babura S R. Determination of carbohydrate and **β-carotene content of some** vegetables consumed in Kano Metropolis, Nigeria. *Bayero Journal of Pure and Applied Sciences.* 2009;2(1):p.119-121.
283. Mustapha P, Babura S R. Determination of carbohydrate and **β-carotene content of some vegetables consumed in Kano Metropolis, Nigeria.** *Bayero Journal of Pure and Applied Sciences.* 2009;2(1):p.119-121.
284. Anwar F, Latif S, Ashraf M, Gilani A H. *Moringa oleifera*: A food plant with multiple medicinal uses. *Phytother Res.* 2007;21:p.17-25.
285. Mahmood K T, Mugal T, Haq I U. *Moringa oleifera*: A natural gift-A review. *J. Pharmac. Sci. Res.* 2010; 2:p.775-781.
286. Tesfay S Z, Bertling I, A O, Workneh T S, Mathaba N. Levels of antioxidants in different parts of moringa
287. (*Moringa oleifera*) seedling. *African Journal of Agricultural Research.* 2011 October 12:6(22):p.5123-5132
288. Kerksick C, Harvey T, Stout J, Campbell B, Wilborn C, Kreider R, Kalman D, Ziegenfuss T, Lopez H, Landis J, Ivy JL, Antonio J: International Society of Sports Nutrition position stand: Nutrient timing. *J Int Soc Sports Nutr* 2008;5:p.17.
289. Anwar F Latif S Ashraf M Gilani A H. *Moringa oleifera*: A food plant with multiple medicinal uses. *Phytother Res.* 2007;21:p.17-25
290. Proske U, Weerakkody N S, Percival P, Morgan D L, Gregory J E, Canny B J. Force-matching errors after eccentric exercise attributed to muscle soreness. Clin and Experimental Pharmacology and Physiology 2003;30: p.576-579.

291. Cleak M J, Eston R. Muscle soreness, swelling, stiffness and strength loss after intense eccentric exercise. *Brit J Sports Med.* 1992; 26:p.267-272.
292. Armstrong R B. Mechanisms of exercise-induced delayed onset muscular soreness: a brief review. *Medicine and Science in Sports and Exercise.* 1984;16:p.529-538.
293. Roth S. Why does lactic acid build up in muscles? And why does it cause soreness? *Scientific American.* 2006;Jan 23:
294. Howatson G, van Someren K A. The prevention and treatment of exercise-induced muscle damage. *Sports Med.* 2008;38(6):p.483-503.
295. Nosaka K, Sacco P, Mawatari K. Effects of amino acid supplementation on muscle soreness and damage. *Int J Sport Nutr Exerc Metab.* 2006;16:p.620-635.
296. Hasson S M, Daniels J C, Divine J G, Niebuhr B R, Richmond S, Stein P G, Williams J H. Effect of ibuprofen use on muscle soreness, damage, and performance: a preliminary investigation. *Med Sci Sports Exerc.* 25:p.9–17.
297. Hasson S M, Daniels J C, Divine J G, Niebuhr B R, Richmond S, Stein P G, Williams J H. Effect of ibuprofen use on muscle soreness, damage, and performance: a preliminary investigation. *Med Sci Sports Exerc.* 25:p.9–17.
298. Cheung K, Hume P, Maxwell L.. Delayed onset muscle soreness: treatment strategies and performance factors. *Sports Medicine.* 2003; 33:p.145-164.
299. Matzke G R. Nonrenal toxicities of acetaminophen, aspirin, and nonsteroidal anti-inflammatory agents. *Am J Kidney Dis.* 1996; 28:p.S63–S70.
300. Trappe T A, White F, Lambert C P, Cesar D, Hellerstein M, Evans W J. Effect of ibuprofen and acetaminophen on post exercise muscle protein synthesis. *Am J Physiol Endocrinol Metab.* 2002;Mar 1(282)(3):p.E551-E556.
301. Fuglie L J. *The Miracle Tree: Moringa oleifera: Natural Nutrition for the Tropics.* Church World Service, Dakar. 1999:68pp.

302. Anwar F, Latif S, Ashraf M, Gilani A H. *Moringa oleifera*: A food plant with multiple medicinal uses. *Phytother Res.* 2007;21:p.17-25.
303. Delaveau P, et al. Oils of *Moringa oleifera* and *Moringa drouhardii*. *Plantes Médicinales et Phytothérapie.* 1980;14(10):p.29-33.
304. Caceres A, Saravia A, Rizzo S, Zabala L, Leon E D, Nave F. Pharmacological properties of *Moringa oleifera*. 2: Screening for antispasmodic, anti-inflammatory and diuretic activity. *J Ethnopharmacol.* 1992;36:p.233-237.
305. Ezeamuzie I C, Ambakederemo A W, Shode F O, Ekwebelm S C. Antiinflammatory effects of *Moringa oleifera* root extract. *Int J Pharmacog.* 1996;34(3):p.207-212.
306. Rao K N V, Gopalakrishnan V, Loganathan V, Shanmuganathan S. Antiinflammatory activity of *Moringa oleifera* Lam. *Ancient Science of Life.* 1999;18(3-4):p.195-198.
307. Udapa S L, Udapa A L, et al. Studies on the anti-inflammatory and wound healing properties of *Moringa oleifera* and Aegle marmelos. *Fitoterapia.* 1994;65(2):p.119-123.
308. Sen C K. Antioxidants in exercise nutrition. *Sports Med.* 2001;31:p.891-908.
309. Watson T A, Callister R, Taylor R D, Sibbritt D W, MacDonald-Wicks L K, Garg M L. Antioxidant restriction and oxidative stress in short-duration exhaustive exercise. *Medicine and Science in Sports and Exercise.* 2005;37(1):p.63-67.
310. Balakrishnan S, Anuradha C. Exercise, depletion of antioxidants and antioxidant manipulation. *Cell Biochem Funct.* 1998;16:p.269-275.
311. Barclay J K, Hansel M. Free radicals may contribute to oxidative skeletal muscle fatigue. *Can J Physiol Pharmacol.* 1991;69:p.279-284.
312. Viguie C A, Frei B, Shigenaga M K, Ames B N, Packer L, Brooks G A. Antioxidant status and indexes of oxidative stress during consecutive days of exercise. *J Appl Physiol.* 1993;75:P.566-572.
313. Cooper C E, Vollaard N B, Choueiri T, Wilson M T. Exercise, free radicals and oxidative stress. *Biochem Soc Trans.* 2002;30:p.280-285.

314. McArdle A, Pattwell D Vasilaki A, Griffiths R D, M. J. Jackson M J.. Contractile activity-induced oxidative stress: cellular origin and adaptive responses. *Am J Physiol Cell Physiol.* 2001;280:p.C621-627.
315. Clarkson P M. Antioxidants and physical performance. *Crit Rev Food Sci Nutr.* 1995;35:p.131-141.
316. Brown E C, DiSilvestro R A, Babaknia A, Devor S T. Soy versus whey protein bars: Effects on exercise training impact on lean body mass and antioxidant status. *Nutr J.* 2004;December 8:p.3-22.
317. Kehrer J. Free radicals as mediators of tissue injury and disease. *Crit Rev Toxicol.* 1993;23:p.21-48.
318. Watson T A, Callister R, Taylor R D, Sibbritt D W, MacDonald-Wicks L K, Garg M L. Antioxidant restriction and oxidative stress in short-duration exhaustive exercise. *Medicine and Science in Sports and Exercise.* 2005;37(1):p.63-67.
319. Supinski G, Nethery D, Stofan D, DiMarco A. Effect of free radical scavengers on diaphragmatic fatigue. *Am J Respir Crit Care Med.* 1997;155:p.622-629.
320. Karlsson J. Antioxidants and Exercise. Champaign IL: Human Kinetics. 1997.
321. McGinley C, Shafat A, Donnelly A. Does antioxidant vitamin supplementation protect against muscle damage? *Sports Med.* 2009;39(12):p1011-1032.
322. Sen C K. Antioxidants in exercise nutrition. *Sports Med.* 2001;31:p.891-908.
323. Kumar N A, Pari I. Antioxidant action of *Moringa oleifera* Lam (drumstick) against antitubercular drug induced lipid peroxidation in rats. *J Medicinal Foods.* 2003;6(3):p.255-259.
324. Bharali R, Tabassum J, Azad M R H. Chemomodulatory effect of *Moringa oleifera*, Lam, on hepatic carcinogen metabolizing enzymes, antioxidant parameters and skin papillomagenesis in mice. *Asian Pacific Journal of Cancer Prevention* 2003;4:p.131-139.
325. Njoku O U, Adikwu M U. Investigation on some physico-chemical antioxidant and toxicological properties of *Moringa oleifera* seed oil. *Acta Pharmaceutica Zagreb.* 1997;47(4): p.87-290.

326. Siddhuraju P, Becker K. Antioxidant properties of various solvent extracts of total phenolic constituents from three different agroclimatic origins of drumstick tree (*Moringa oleifera* Lam.) leaves. *Journal of Agricultural and Food Chemistry.* 2003;51:p.2144-2155.
327. DiSilvestro R A. Antioxidant actions of soya. *Food Indust J.* 2001;4:p.210-220.
328. DiSilvestro R A. Antioxidant actions of soya. *Food Indust J.* 2001;4:p.210-220.
329. Lalas S, Tsaknis J. Extraction & identification of natural antioxidant from the seeds of *Moringa oleifera* tree of Malavi. *J A. Oil Chemists Soc.* 2002;79(7):p.677-683.
330. Kehrer J. Free radicals as mediators of tissue injury and disease. *Crit Rev Toxicol.* 1993;23:p.21-48.
331. Blackburn E, Greider C W, Szostack J W. Telomeres and telomerase: The path from maize, *Tetrahymena* and yeast to human cancer and aging. *Nature Medicine.* 2006;12:p.1133-1138.
332. Schippinger G, Wonisch W, Abuja P M, Fankhauser F, Winklhofer-Roob B M, Halwachs G. Lipid peroxidation and antioxidant status in professional American football players during competition. *Eur J Clin Invest.* 2002;32:p.686-692.
333. Bergholm R, Makimattila S, Valkonen M, Liu ML, Lahdenpera S, Taskinen MR, Sovijarvi A, Malmberg P, Yki-Jarvinen H. Intense physical training decreases circulating antioxidants and endothelium-dependent vasodilatation in vivo. *Atherosclerosis.* 1999;145:341-349
334. Kehrer J. Free radicals as mediators of tissue injury and disease. *Crit Rev Toxicol.* 1993;23:p.21-48.
335. Kumar N A, Pari I. Antioxidant action of *Moringa oleifera* Lam (drumstick) against antitubercular drug induced lipid peroxidation in rats. *J Medicinal Foods.* 2003;6(3):p.255-259.
336. Fakurazi S, U. Nanthini U, Hairuszah I, 2008. Hepatoprotective and Antioxidant Action of *Moringa oleifera* Lam.Against

Acetaminophen Induced Hepatotoxicity in Rats. *International Journal of Pharmacology*, 2008;4: 270-275.
337. DiSilvestro R A. Antioxidant actions of soya. *Food Indust J.* 2001;4:p.210-220.
338. Fahey J W. *Moringa oleifera*: a review of the medical evidence for its nutritional, therapeutic, and prophylactic properties. *Trees for Life Journal.* 2005;1(5) p. 1-13.
339. Kerksick C, Harvey T, Stout J, Campbell B, Wilborn C, Kreider R, Kalman D, Ziegenfuss T, Lopez H, Landis J, Ivy JL, Antonio J: International Society of Sports Nutrition position stand: Nutrient timing. *J Int Soc Sports Nutr* 2008;5:p.17.
340. Tang J E, Manolakos J J, Kujbida G W, Lysecki P J, Moore D R, Phillips S M. Minimal whey protein with carbohydrate stimulates muscle protein synthesis following resistance exercise in trained young men. *Appl Physiol Nutr Metab.* 2007;32:p.1132-1138
341. Haff G G, Lehmkuhl M J, McCoy L B, Stone M H. Carbohydrate supplementation and resistance training. *J StrengthCond Res.* 2003; Feb 17(1):p.187-196.
342. Hulmi J J, Kovanen V, Selänne H, Kraemer WJ, Häkkinen K, Mero A A. Acute and long-term effects of resistance exercise with or without protein ingestion on muscle hypertrophy and gene expression. *Amino Acids* 2009, 37:p.297-308.
343. Gibala M J. Nutritional supplementation and resistance exercise:what is the evidence for enhanced skeletal muscle hypertrophy? *Can J Appl Physioli.* 2000;Dec 25(6):p.524-535.
344. NIH Record. NIH Celebrates Earth Day 2008. Vol LX. No.6. March 21, 2008. http://nihrecord.od.nih.gov/newsletters/2008/03_21_2008/story4.htm
345. Duke J. Duke's ethanobotanical and phytochemistry database. 1998; www.arsgrin.gov/duke/.
346. The Westminster Confession of Faith.(Free Presbyterian Press, 1995) pg. 287-288.

ABOUT THE AUTHOR

Dr. Howard Fisher specializes in Anti-Aging medicine from a natural perspective and is on a mission to educate and enlighten the world about the toxic factors that exist in our environment and their direct relationship to our health. His current seminar that he delivers to both Medical Anti-Aging Conferences and Health Conferences world-wide, makes both professionals and the public aware of the omnipresent threats present in our immediate environment and gives insightful plans for remediation. Dr. Fisher lectures internationally on anti-aging, nutrition, wellness, and immunology. He has written many articles for trade publications and is a featured guest on many radio and television broadcasts. In addition to authoring twenty health-oriented books, his research has also been published in peer-reviewed journals. His books and lectures have been translated into seven languages and are sold in North America, Europe, and Asia.

Being widely recognized for his ability to easily assimilate what many view as daunting scientific and clinical information, Dr. Fisher transforms essential knowledge that would otherwise remain inaccessible to the public into readily available life-altering information. The foundation of his philosophy rests upon understanding and exposing the true nutritional and environmental deficiencies that exist in our everyday lives, and scouring the planet for the most efficient solutions to not only solving these threatening health issues, but improving the well-being and overall quality of life for everyone. His common sense approach to explaining the impact of our environmental factors on the health of the world makes it easy for his audience to make informed choices towards bettering their lives.

In addition to his research, writing, and lecturing, Dr. Fisher is still an avid athlete who runs, plays hockey, and can be found on the golf course most mornings. A dynamic and colorful personality, Dr. Fisher resides in Toronto, Ontario with his wife and two children when not lecturing abroad.

OTHER BOOKS BY DR. HOWARD W. FISHER

Wisdom of the Woods: Herbal Remedies

Extreme Toxic Times: How to Escape On Your Own Two Feet

Reishi Rescue: R & R for Your Immune System

Before You Breathe Deeply: The Immunological Significance of Breathing Purified Air

Nature's Silver Bullet: Killing the Fear Factor

Reishi Response: Answering Today's Health Challenges

Approaching Wellness: Simple Steps to Restore Your Immune System

Enzymes and Your Health: Optimizing Your Physiological Functions

The Invisible Threat : The Risks Associated With EMFs

The Invisible Threat II: A Solution to the EMF Radiation Crisis.

Molecular Resonance Effect Technology: The Dynamic Effects on Human Physiology

Optimal Hydration the Key to Health and Anti-Aging

Moringa Oleifera: Magic, Myth or Miracle

In Pursuit of Perfection: *Moringa Oleifera*, The Peak Performance Partner